A Nurse's Survival Guide to Primary Care

Neither the publishers nor the author will be liable for any loss or damage of any nature occasioned to or suffered by any person acting or refraining from acting as a result of reliance on the material contained in this publication.

For Churchill Livingstone:

Senior commissioning editor: Alex Mathieson
Project manager: Ewan Halley
Project development editor: Valerie Dearing
Design direction: Judith Wright
Project controller: Jane Shanks

A Nurse's Survival Guide to Primary Care

Rosemary Cook MSc RGN PNCert
Manager, Manchester Multi-disciplinary Audit and Quality
Group, Manchester, UK

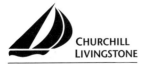

CHURCHILL LIVINGSTONE

EDINBURGH LONDON NEW YORK PHILADELPHIA
SYDNEY TORONTO 1999

CHURCHILL LIVINGSTONE

Churchill Livingstone, Robert Stevenson House, 1–3 Baxter's Place,
Leith Walk, Edinburgh EH1 3AF, UK

First published 1999

ISBN 0 443 06115 7

British Library Cataloguing in Publication Data
A catalogue record for this book is available from the British Library.

Library of Congress Cataloging in Publication Data
A catalog record for this book is available from the Library of
Congress.

Note
Medical knowledge is constantly changing. As new information
becomes available, changes in treatment, procedures, equipment and
the use of drugs become necessary. The author and the publishers
have, as far as it is possible, taken care to ensure that the information
given in this text is accurate and up-to-date. However, readers are
strongly advised to confirm that the information, especially with
regard to drug usage, complies with the latest legislation and
standards of practice.

The
publisher's
policy is to use
**paper manufactured
from sustainable forests**

Printed in China
EPC/01

CONTENTS

PREFACE

This book is an introduction to primary care, aimed primarily at nursing students getting their first experiences of nursing outside hospital settings.

The book aims to do three things: first, to paint a broad-brush picture of primary care, showing how the community, general practice, nursing homes and other settings are interwoven with each other and with society as a whole to provide the context for primary health care; second, to bring together some of the policy changes and professional developments which shape everyday health care and nursing practice; and third, to highlight some of the many different areas of clinical practice in primary care, giving practical ideas for applying the nursing principles and clinical experience gained elsewhere in the particular settings of primary care.

It will not, however, tell you all you need to know to nurse in primary care; there are too many variables – different settings, different professionals, different patient circumstances – to allow for prescriptive guidance on 'what to do'. Details of nursing procedures, drug regimes, or anatomy and physiology are not generally included in this book. There are many more detailed texts which cover these topics, and many clinical experts working in primary care who can contribute to the development of the necessary clinical skills.

There are two ways to use this book. One way is to read through the first two sections to learn something of the 'big picture' of primary care. The way that nurses are employed, the work they do, where they do it and what career opportunities are available to them, are all dependent on health policy, health service structure and professional developments. The experiences of patients, the quality of care available to them, and their health or ill health, also depend on all these things. These things cannot be ignored. Today more than ever, nurses need to understand the context in which they work, in order to fulfil the basic professional requirement to safeguard and promote the interests of individual patients and clients. The other way to use this book is to dip into the later sections as you prepare to become involved in the different areas of work covered. You won't necessarily find a checklist of right answers but there will be guidance on the scope of nurses' work in the area, and ways to apply your professional principles and skills to the very different world of primary care.

In acute care, patients can sometimes be viewed as if through the wrong end of a telescope: their disease looms large, and their real life shrinks into the background. In primary care, the background is life-size, and illness, the threat of illness, and harmful behaviour, are simply features of the landscape. Working with people, by influence and empowerment, building relationships which enable them to receive care when they need it, and acting as advocates for them when they need more than the care we can give, is what makes nursing in primary care a skill and a challenge.

Rosemary Cook 1998

SECTION 1

Background to primary care

1

What is 'primary care'?

Nurses who have been working in hospital settings, or who have only recently entered the profession, may not be familiar with the use of the term 'primary care' as a setting for nursing care. Terms like nursing 'in the community' or 'on the district' are more familiar descriptions of nursing which takes place in patients' homes, or other places away from the traditional hospital ward or clinic.

The most familiar roles in the community in the past have probably been those of district nurses and health visitors. But recent Government policy changes, changes to the technology of health care and to people's demands and expectations, have led to a rapid and prodigious expansion of the health services provided outside of hospital settings. To deliver these services, there have been equally dramatic and significant changes to the roles of nurses and other professionals. There are more opportunities for nurses to work in more innovative and challenging roles in primary care than ever before.

It is not only the everyday work of nurses, health visitors and others which defines primary care. There are also broad policy issues which cut across the work of every individual professional in primary care, and have a direct impact on what they do and how they do it (see Figure 1.1). To take a narrow view, confined to one branch of the profession and its particular concerns, is to miss the opportunity to see one's professional work in context, and understand the 'how' and 'why' as well as the 'what' of one's role.

> ⚠ **For nurses to act both as advocates for patients in a modern-day health service, and as accountable practitioners within their profession, it is necessary for them to have a clear understanding of the 'bigger picture'.**

TERMINOLOGY

The term 'primary care' is used in many different ways. This section looks at some of these usages, and explores alternative definitions. The way that the term 'primary care' is used in this book is explained.

THE WORLD HEALTH ORGANIZATION VIEW

There are many different definitions of primary care. Twenty years ago, the World Health Organization produced one of the most commonly cited, and certainly most comprehensive, definitions of primary care:

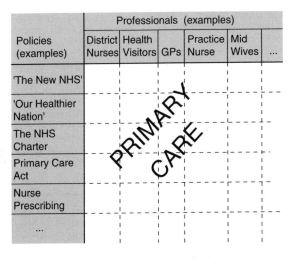

Policies (examples)	Professionals (examples)					
	District Nurses	Health Visitors	GPs	Practice Nurse	Mid Wives	...
'The New NHS'						
'Our Healthier Nation'						
The NHS Charter						
Primary Care Act						
Nurse Prescribing						
...						

Fig 1.1 The interface of professional policy issues in primary care.

> '...essential health care based on practical, scientifically sound and socially acceptable methods and technology, made universally available to individuals and families in the community through their full participation and at a cost that the community and the country can afford to maintain at every stage of their development in the spirit of self-reliance and self-determination' (WHO 1978).

This definition is deliberately complex and broad, as it relates to all countries and encompasses international perspectives on health care. As such it may not be helpful to the nurse trying to determine what primary care is in practical terms in the context of the National Health Service in the UK. Another part of this 'Alma Ata Declaration' (named after the venue of the Conference in the former USSR) described primary care as:

> **'the first level of contact of individuals, the family, and the community with the national health system, bringing health care as close as possible to where people live and work'.**

This briefer description is a more useful and usable guide to what constitutes primary care in the UK. The 'first level of contact' with the health service is usually through a person's general practitioner (who refers on to a hospital service or consultant if necessary), practice nurse (based in the general practitioner's (GP's) surgery), health visitor or other professional such as a dietitian to whom the public have direct access. All these professionals, and others, are part of the primary health care team (see next chapter), and therefore of primary care. 'Bringing health care as close as possible to where people live and work' identifies primary care as the services delivered in people's homes, by district nurses and health visitors, for example; in local health centres and surgeries by GPs, practice nurses, dietitians, counsellors and others; and in places of work such as factories, schools and shops by occupational health nurses and school nurses.

OTHER VIEWS

It has been said that the WHO definition represents 'more of a description of a desirable state of affairs than a concrete definition on which to base any plans to develop a primary health care system' (Vuori 1986). Vuori proposes that the term 'primary care' can be used to mean four different things:

- a set of activities
- a level of care
- a strategy for organizing health services
- a philosophy that should permeate the entire health system.

Activities

In the National Health Service (NHS) primary care system, these activities would include among other things community nursing, childhood immunization programmes, GP services, community dental practitioner services, and pharmacy services. This definition would also include activities aimed at maintaining the health of the population which are not solely or mainly the responsibility of the health service, but on which health care professionals may collaborate with other services, such as local authorities.

> **⚠ Examples of these are the provision of clean, safe water supplies and sanitation, and the maintenance of clean air and a safer environment.**

Level of care

This refers to the 'first contact' concept: primary care is the first port of call for people with health needs or concerns. 'Secondary care' therefore refers to services which come later in the patient's experience, after referral from their first point of contact. An example is hospital inpatient or outpatient care, following referral from a GP.

Strategy

The Department of Health adopted a strategy of a 'primary-care led NHS' in the 1990s, with White Papers such as 'Primary Care – Choice and Opportunities', 'Primary Care – the Future' and 'Delivering the Future' in 1996, and 'The New NHS – Modern, Dependable' in 1997. Although there is no single definition of this strategy, it refers generally to measures designed to develop health services close to the patient rather than in hospitals, and to involve primary care professionals such as GPs and community nurses in the planning and commissioning of health services.

Philosophy

> ⚠️ 'A country can claim to practise primary health care only if its entire health care system is characterized by social justice and equality, international solidarity, self-responsibility and an acceptance of the broad definition of health' (Vuori 1986).

A GP'S VIEW

Donald Pereira Gray, writing in a paper published by the Royal College of General Practitioners (1992), gives a GP's view of the aims of primary care. They are:

- to diagnose, treat and manage common and chronic illness
- to refer appropriately to specialist care and to manage patients after discharge from specialist care
- to actively promote the health of people through screening, immunization, family planning and health education
- to reassure the worried well
- to provide a choice of doctor and practice
- to be accessible
- to offer a range of professional skills.

Identifying services which fulfil these aims is one way of defining what constitutes primary care in the UK.

DIFFERENTIATING PRIMARY CARE

The following checklist identifies the features which make

primary care different from specialist (or secondary) care (Fry et al 1995).

Long-term, continuing, comprehensive and coordinated care
A health visitor, for example, may have a family on his/her caseload for a number of years, and provide advice, education and support on a range of issues from parenting skills and immunization to housing problems and bereavement, identifying health needs and coordinating other professionals and services as necessary.

Access/availability GPs have 24 hour responsibility for their registered patients: if they do not take 'out of hours' calls themselves, they must ensure that another doctor is available to their patients. Other professionals in primary care offer direct access to patients: that is, patients can refer themselves without needing to see their GP first. *Examples are district continence advisors, family planning nurses, occupational health nurses and practice nurses.*

First-contact care Primary care is the patient's first port of call when they need, or may need, health care.

Population basis This is one of the most important differences between primary and secondary care. Primary care is based on the dual concept of delivering services to *individuals* who are part of a larger *population*. This may be a list of registered patients, such as a GP's patients; or the population of a health district, regardless of which GP they are registered with; or a population defined by age (e.g. children under 5 years) or physical condition (e.g. pregnant women). *District continence advisors or community diabetic specialist nurses work with the whole population of a district, including every age group, while community paediatric nurses' services focus on children with specific health needs.*

PRIMARY CARE IN THE UK HEALTH SERVICE

Clearly there is a lengthy and wide-ranging debate about the meaning of primary care, and many different ways of describing this sector of health care. In the UK, however, the term 'primary care' is often used in a pragmatic way, rather than a philosophical one, to describe one part of the health service. Unfortunately, there is not always agreement about which part of the health service it should be used to describe.

'Primary care' is sometimes used to mean only primary *medical* care: that is, GP services. Alongside this usage of the term 'primary care' comes the use of the term 'community', as in 'community nursing' or patients being treated 'in the community', to describe the work of district nurses, health visitors and others working outside of acute hospitals. The

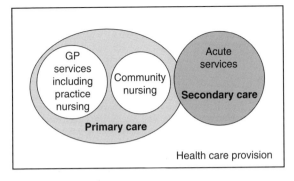

Fig 1.2 Primary and secondary health care.

whole arena of care outside the acute sector then has to be described rather clumsily as 'primary and community care', in order to include both of these parts.

In a simpler version of the term 'primary care', which is becoming increasingly common, it is used to mean GP services, community nursing services, as well as services provided by the professions allied to medicine (PAMs) and others. In this case it refers to all health care services provided outside of the acute hospital sector, by all the health care professionals, and sometimes others, such as social workers, too. Acute care services are then referred to as 'secondary care', to differentiate them from primary care. (See Figure 1.2.)

> ⚠ **This broader definition of primary care does not exclude some forms of institutional care. Patients may be inpatients in a nursing home or continuing care hospital, but still be in primary care under the care of their GP and primary health care team.**

Throughout this book, the term primary care is used in this broad sense to mean all health care, including prevention and health promotion, which takes place in settings outside of acute hospitals, including patient's homes, and is provided by GPs, nurses, health visitors, PAMs and others.

ORGANIZATION OF PRIMARY CARE

In order to understand the structure and functioning of primary care in the UK health service, it is essential to

Primary care in the UK health service   What is 'primary care'?

9

understand how the different parts of the NHS are constituted, and how they relate to each other. The following brief overview outlines the context in which primary care nursing has taken place in the years since the beginning of the NHS.

1948

The basis of the NHS was proposed in the Beveridge Report of 1942, and the service was set up in 1948 by the National Health Service Act of 1946. The Act extended the established national health insurance principles, which already covered half of the UK population, to the whole population. The founding principles of the NHS, which have been reiterated through the many organizational changes in subsequent years, were:

- equity – the right of every person to receive equal care for equal need
- comprehensiveness – the service to address all health care needs
- services free at the point of delivery – paid for through national insurance and income tax contributions.

The effect of the nationalized service was to make the state both the funder and provider of health care, a model which lasted for more than forty years.

In this early model of the health service, community nursing services – district nursing (sometimes also called domicillary nursing, because the care is delivered in the patient's home) and health visiting – were the responsibility of local authorities, not health authorities. General practitioners remained independent contractors, not employed by the NHS, but providing services to it under contracts administered by Executive Councils (see Chapter 4).

So primary care at this time was fragmented into three distinct entities:

- independent general practice, providing general medical services under contract
- community nursing, managed by local authorities
- the overall service management of health services, which rested with the health authorities.

Although health visitors and district nurses were employed by local authorities, the establishment of health centres and health clinics which began in the 1960s meant that they were sometimes able to work in close proximity to GP practices, in spite of the organizational fragmentation which separated them.

1965

The Charter for the Family Doctor Service, which came into effect in 1965, gave GPs financial help to employ practice staff, including nurses. From this time there was an increase in the numbers of nurses directly employed by GPs, and so working in primary care. At this time they tended to be 'treatment room nurses', working solely in GP premises, rather than in patients' homes or clinics like other community nurses.

1974

The first major structural reorganization of the NHS took place in 1974. It was intended to rationalize the management of the service, and created three tiers of authority: Regional Health Authorities, Area Health Authorities, and District Health Authorities. The bodies administering GPs' contracts changed from Executive Councils to Family Practitioner Committees (see Figure 1.3) but remained separate from health authorities. A major effect of this reorganization was to bring community nursing services under the remit of health authorities instead of local authorities, laying the organizational groundwork for primary health care teams (see Chapter 3).

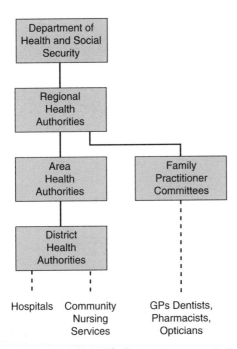

Fig 1.3 Structure of the NHS after the 1974 reorganization.

1982

1982 brought a second major reorganization of the NHS. Area Health Authorities were abolished, leaving Regional and District Health Authorities to finance and provide health services using their allocation of the NHS funding (see Figure 1.4).

1990s

The most significant reforms of the organization and financing of the health service took place in the 1990s. A series of White Papers including 'Promoting Better Health' (1987), 'Caring for People' (1989) and 'Working for Patients' (1989) proposed some major reforms for the health service as a whole, and in particular for primary care. The NHS and Community Care Act, 1990, provided the statutory basis for these changes.

At the same time, a new GP Contract was introduced in 1990, making some of the most radical changes in that arena since 1965. Among the many changes introduced by this combination of reforms were measures designed to increase emphasis on:

- disease prevention and health promotion
- a primary-care-led NHS
- consumer participation in health care
- needs assessment and priority setting

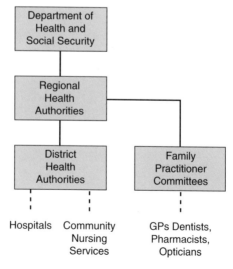

Fig 1.4 Structure of the NHS after the 1982 reorganization.

- flexibility of services
- clinical audit.

The internal market The single most radical change introduced at this time was the separation of the purchasing and providing functions in the health service. Sometimes referred to as the 'purchaser–provider split', or the introduction of an 'internal market' in health care, this fundamentally altered the way the health service was run, and had a direct impact on community nursing. Before this reform, district health authorities (DHAs) had been responsible for financing *and* providing health care in their districts. They had managed the hospitals and community clinics within their boundaries and employed the staff who worked in them (the 'providing' function), as well as planning and financing new services and facilities for their district population (the 'purchasing' function).

The effect of the internal market, introduced from 1 April 1991, was to split the functions of providing, which were now to be carried out by the hospitals and community units, and purchasing, to be carried out by the District Health Authorities (see Figure 1.5).

In the internal market, the responsibilities of the District Health Authorities, as purchasers, were:

- to assess the health needs of their populations
- to commission health services to meet those needs from 'providers'

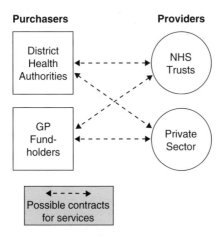

Fig 1.5 The 'internal market' in health care, following the 1990 reforms.

• to purchase the appropriate services through contracts with providers, using finance allocated for their District.

The responsibilities of the hospitals and community units, as 'providers', were:

• to deliver care to patients as specified in their contracts with purchasers,
• to employ professional and other staff in order to do so. These hospital and community units were to become NHS 'Trusts', self-governing bodies competing with each other for contracts from purchasers, in order to generate the income necessary to pay staff, maintain buildings and develop services. The reforms also allowed for private providers (i.e. other than NHS Trusts) to bid for contracts with purchasers, so introducing another element of competition into the market.

GP fundholding The other major innovation of the 1990 reforms was the introduction of GP fundholding. This allowed general practices which fulfilled certain criteria of size and management capability to opt to hold a budget with which they could purchase some of the services necessary for their registered patient population. They negotiated with provider Trusts in the same way as the health authority purchasers, and contracted for services of the appropriate quantity and quality for their patients.

Initially, fundholders were restricted to purchasing a limited range of secondary care services, as well as holding a budget for the drugs they prescribed and the staff they employed. Later expansions in the scope of fundholding, and in the criteria for entering the scheme, encouraged more practices to take part, and to purchase a wider range of services. By 1996, over half the GPs in England and Wales had joined the scheme, and a range of different forms of fundholding were in action (see Chapter 4).

As fundholding GPs continued to provide general medical services to their patients, whilst purchasing other services–including secondary care and (from 1993) community nursing services – they were in effect fulfilling a dual role as purchasers and providers. GPs who opted not to hold their own budgets had services purchased for their patients by their local DHA.

From 1996, the DHAs and the Family Health Services Authorities (FHSAs) were replaced by new Health Authorities (HAs). The new authorities combined the commissioning and purchasing responsibilities of the former DHAs with the administration of GPs' and other independent practitioners' contracts which had been the FHSAs' responsibility. This final piece of the internal market jigsaw is illustrated in Figure 1.6.

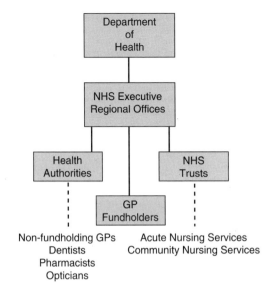

Non-fundholding GPs   Acute Nursing Services
Dentists   Community Nursing Services
Pharmacists
Opticians

Fig 1.6 The NHS after the creation of new Health Authorities in 1996.

The effects on community nursing   All nurses in primary care found their role and work changing as a result of this wave of policy activity:

• There was increased emphasis on preventive activities and screening clinics, brought about by the GP Contract and by the health strategy document 'The Health of the Nation' published in 1992 (see Chapter 12).
• The targets set for health promotion, cervical cytology and child immunization in the GP Contract brought a rapid increase in the numbers of practice nurses employed, and changed their role from treatment room nurses to include health promotion and the management of screening and prevention programmes (see Chapter 2).
• An increase in day surgery and hospital at home schemes, aiming to keep people in their own homes for as long as possible and so increase the capacity of the provider hospitals, meant that district nurses and community paediatric nurses were dealing with more dependent patients in more acute stages of illness or recovery.

But for the traditional community nursing specialisms of district nursing and health visiting, there was a more fundamental change. The major effect of these reforms on community nursing was to make it a service to be purchased by contract, rather than simply an arena for professional practice. Nurses and health visitors working in primary care have been made aware of this in a very practical way, since, in order to define the service which purchasers are paying for, their activity is currently measured by the number of 'contacts' they make with patients or clients. The contract between the health authority or GP purchaser specifies the number of contacts they expect for the payment they make to the employing Trust. It is generally recognized, however, that counting contacts alone fails to recognize the value of much of the work that is carried out with individuals, families and communities. Some Trusts and purchasers are trying to develop an alternative measure for these services, but in the mean time, 'contacts' remains a measure of quantity rather than of quality of service.

Some fundholding GPs, in their role as purchasers, have reviewed the work of the nurses and health visitors employed by the Trust to see how the community nursing service dovetails with the work carried out by their directly-employed practice nurses. In some cases this has led to more integrated nursing teams (see Chapter 3). In others it has led GPs to question the need to purchase community nursing and especially health visiting services in the same quantity as before.

1997
The Secretary of State for Health's White Paper 'The New NHS – Modern, Dependable', published in 1997, announced the end of the internal market. The plans intend to replace the competition generated by the market with cooperation and 'integrated care', and to set up primary care groups, led by GPs and community nurses, to assess health needs of local communities and to commission health care to meet those needs. The primary care groups, as well as health authorities, Trusts and local authorities, will draw up and work to a local Health Improvement Programme.

Ultimately, 'primary care Trusts' will be set up which will provide all community nursing services and run community hospitals, as well as commissioning secondary care. These changes should have the effect of unifying the GP service and community nursing to a greater degree than ever before.

SUMMARY

It is important for nurses working in primary care to have a clear understanding of the 'bigger picture': of the structure, policies and politics of the health service. Each of these elements has a direct influence on the way nurses are able to work, on the exercise of their professional accountability for the care they give, and on their personal circumstances such as employment conditions and pensions. The proposals set out in 'The New NHS' White Paper will enable nurses to take part for the first time in the planning and commissioning of care for people.

References

Department of Health and Social Security 1987 Promoting better health: the Government's programme for improving primary health care. HMSO, London

Department of Health 1989 Working for patients. HMSO, London

Department of Health 1989 Caring for people: community care in the next decade and beyond. HMSO, London

Department of Health 1992 The health of the nation: a strategy of health for England. HMSO, London

Department of Health 1996 Primary care: choice and opportunities. HMSO, London

Department of Health 1996 Primary care: the future. HMSO, London

Department of Health 1996 Primary care: delivering the future. HMSO, London

Department of Health 1997 The new NHS–modern, dependable. The Stationery Office, London

Fry J, Light D, Rodnick J, Orton P 1995 Reviving primary care–a UK/US comparison. Radcliffe Medical Press, Oxford

Pereira Gray D 1992 Planning primary care; RCGP Occasional Paper 57. Royal College of General Practitioners, London

Vuori H 1986 'Health for all, primary health care and general practitioners' [keynote address]. WONCA, 1986

WHO 1978 Report of the international conference on primary health care, Alma Ata, USSR, 6–12 September 1978. World Health Organization, Geneva

Further reading

Leathard A 1990 Health care provision–past present and future. Chapman and Hall, London

Baggott R 1998 Health and health care in Britain, 2nd edn. Macmillan, London

Littlewood J, ed. 1995 Current issues in community nursing–primary health care in practice. Churchill Livingstone, Edinburgh

2

Who's who in primary care

INTRODUCTION

There are many different groups of professionals and others who deliver care in a variety of ways in a primary care setting. One way of distinguishing them would be to divide them into the statutory (e.g. health and social services' workers) and the non-statutory (e.g. voluntary and private sector workers). Another would be to divide the professionals (nurses, doctors, midwives) from the non-professionals (social workers, volunteers). However, for the purposes of this chapter, some of the many different groups and agencies have been set in a model based loosely on their different spheres of activity (see Figure 2.1).

WHO'S WHO

The inner, 'core' team is based around a GP practice population of 'registered' patients. It includes the GP-employed practice nurse, the health visitors, district nurses and other Trust nurses 'attached' to that practice.

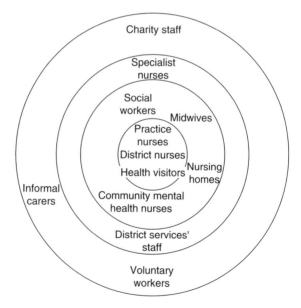

Fig 2.1 A model of some care and nursing services in primary care.

Beyond this team are professionals and others who have a 'patch' or geographical area which usually covers more than one practice: these may include social workers, community mental health nurses, Macmillan nurses and midwives. Nurses working in nursing homes, and occupational health nurses working in industry, also provide care to a defined population, but one defined by their residence or employment, respectively.

Further out are services provided by people with a district-wide remit, such as the diabetes specialist nurse, and the tissue viability specialist.

And, in the outer circle, are the voluntary sector and informal carers who often provide the majority of care to people with chronic or terminal illness.

THE NATURE OF CARE PROVISION

The distinction between health-related care (such as medication, treatment and rehabilitation) and social care (such as help with bathing, adaptations to the home and assistance with benefits claims) is often blurred in primary care. Many people living with chronic disease, or recovering from more acute illnesses at home, require a complex network of such services, delivered by a range of different people working for several different services. In effect, they require a slice of the care cake, incorporating all the different ingredients, rather than moving in a linear fashion into and out of the central core (see Figure 2.2).

> ⚠ **The coordination of such 'packages of care' is one of the challenges of working in a primary care setting.**

This chapter will look at the range of people and agencies involved in delivering primary care, and then explore in more detail the history, work and inter-relationships of some of the primary care nurses, and health visitors.

THE WIDER PICTURE: INFORMAL CARERS

Many of the people involved in caring for patients in primary care are not nurses, nor even members of any of the health care professions. By far the largest part of the 'workforce' comprises the unpaid, informal carers: families, parents,

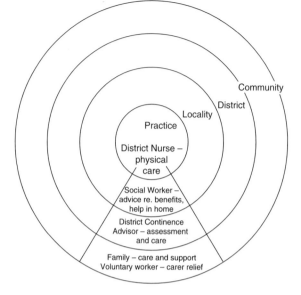

Fig 2.2 An example of a package of care for an individual patient.

partners, friends and neighbours. They provide the majority of care, with the support and specialized input of the primary health care team.

> ⚠ In cases of chronic ill health or terminal illness, it is frequently the informal carers who make the difference between a person's being able to remain in their own home, and needing to be admitted to hospital for care.

Even in more acute situations, the trend for earlier discharge from hospital, and day case surgery, means that informal carers now provide a lot of the early care, following surgical operations and acute illness, that would once have been undertaken by nurses in hospital. It is important to realize that these carers are not necessarily the 'healthy' looking after the 'sick'. Carers themselves may be in poor health, or suffer accidents or illnesses, and sometimes, especially in the case of carers of very elderly people, they may themselves be in later years. Carers groups can provide support, information and sometimes a period of respite from caring, but carers' own health needs have to be recognized and met if they are to be able to continue contributing to the care of the 'original' patient.

THE VOLUNTARY SECTOR

There are numerous voluntary sector or charitable organizations, fulfilling a range of roles from the provision of information, support and contacts, to participating in the day to day care of seriously ill patients in their own homes. Three examples give an indication of the diversity and scope of such services:

The Marie Curie Nursing Service provides an evening and night-sitting service from nurses who are able to give regular carers a chance to sleep, or take a break from caring.

Body Positive is an organization for people living with or affected by the human immunodeficiency virus (HIV). As well as running support groups which care for sufferers and their friends and partners, they organize a 'buddy' system which links each client with a volunteer worker. The volunteer may accompany the client to hospital appointments, assist with personal care, and form a link to other services such as housing departments and social services.

The Royal National Institute for the Deaf (RNID) provides information for deaf people and raises funds for research. In addition they offer advice to professionals who will come into contact with deaf people on the best way to make their service as well as their premises more accessible to the deaf. For example, they have a checklist of measures which can be instituted at a doctor's surgery or health centre to make it easier for a deaf person to use the service effectively and with the minimum of distress or embarrassment. They also provide 'deaf awareness' training to health professionals.

THE PRIVATE SECTOR: NURSING AND RESIDENTIAL HOMES

The Nursing and Residential Care Homes Act of 1984 set out definitions of these two types of private care institutions. Residential homes, which are registered with local authorities, cannot employ registered nurses to provide nursing care. Therefore they can only accommodate residents who require no more care than can be provided by, for example, district nursing services, as if the resident was in his or her own home.

Nursing homes, however, are registered with the health authority, and have to employ registered nurses at a staff: patient ratio set by the health authority. Community nurses may have considerable input into residential homes, providing assessment and care on the same basis as for any person living in their own home. They are also often involved in a multi-agency assessment of the care needs of a client to determine whether they can be appropriately accommodated in a residential, or their own, home, or whether they require hospital or nursing home care.

Another element of the private sector is nursing and home care agencies, which may supply nurses to GP practices as cover for practice nurses, as well as to nursing homes and private individuals.

Occupational health nurses, employed by private companies to provide health screening, treatment and advice to their workforces, and school nurses employed by private schools, are also part of the private sector in primary care.

DISTRICT-WIDE SERVICES: CLINICAL NURSE SPECIALISTS

Each health district will have a range of clinical nurse specialists (CNSs) whose remit includes acting as a resource to their nursing, medical and other colleagues across the district. They therefore cross the 'boundaries' between different GP practices, between different professions and, often, between primary and secondary care. Examples of the clinical areas in which such nurses commonly practice are:

- continence
- palliative care
- breast care
- diabetes
- tissue viability
- stoma care
- HIV/Aids, and others.

In some parts of the country there are clinical nurse specialists in epilepsy, Parkinson's disease and asthma: though these are less common than those listed above.

Outreach
The CNSs may be based – physically, in terms of their office space, or managerially, in terms of their line manager accountability – in primary care, or in secondary care. If they are based in secondary care, but have a remit to advise colleagues in primary care and visit patients in their own homes or in clinics, then this is termed an 'outreach' service. A common example of this model is the HIV/Aids clinical

nurse specialist, who both works on the wards where their clients are treated as inpatients, and works with the district nurse to deliver care to the individual when he/she is at home. The advantages of such an arrangement are the continuity of contact and care experienced by the client, and the availability of the experience and skills of the clinical nurse specialist to the community nurse. It should also minimize the problem of poor communication across the primary/secondary care interface which is so often reported.

Inreach

When the clinical nurse specialist is based in primary care, but also follows clients into hospital when they are receiving inpatient care, to liaise with hospital staff and prepare for the client's eventual discharge, this is termed an 'inreach' service. This has been less common than outreach services, but one specialized example is the 'domino' system (an abbreviated form of 'domicillary in and out') in which a woman is accompanied into hospital by her community midwife for the delivery of her baby, then returns home within a matter of hours to continue receiving care by the same midwife.

Common duties

Whether they are considered inreach or outreach, most clinical nurse specialists will work closely with nursing, medical and other colleagues in both primary and secondary care to ensure that an effective and seamless service is maintained. In order to achieve this, the CNS may:

- visit the patient to assist in the assessment and care planning process
- share some of the delivery of care with other nurses in primary care
- provide advice on an ad hoc basis when requested to do so by nursing colleagues or the patient's GP
- run study days and updating sessions to share specialized knowledge and skills with community colleagues
- work with medical and nursing colleagues from primary and secondary care to produce, disseminate, implement and evaluate protocols or clinical guidelines relating to the condition or client group
- undertake audit of services or carry out research in their specialist field.

GEOGRAPHICALLY BASED SERVICES

There are many examples of professionals whose area of responsibility is based on a geographical area – sometimes called a patch, zone, neighbourhood or locality – rather than the whole of a health district. These may vary from area to area, but some common examples are midwives, social workers, community mental health nurses, community paediatric nurses, physiotherapists and school nurses (who may have a number of schools in one area for which they are responsible).

There are advantages and disadvantages to a patch-based system, for both the professional and the patient or client. The advantages are:

• The professional can develop a detailed knowledge of their patch, both geographically, demographically and in terms of resources, facilities and people.
• It minimizes travelling time (and costs to their employer) as all visits are carried out in the same area.
• People get to know 'their' professionals by being aware of their contact with others in the community.

The disadvantages are:

• Additional time and travel may be involved in professionals' receiving referrals from and liaising with a number of different GPs and primary health care teams, in different surgeries or health centres, as people in their patch will be registered with a range of different practices.
• It is difficult for patch-based professionals to develop effective teamworking with a large number of GPs and primary health care teams, and this can lead to duplication of effort and poor communication.

Most community Trusts have now implemented 'attachment' of district nurses and health visitors to one or more GP practices, to overcome these two major disadvantages of the patch-based system.

Although not employed by the GP, these professionals work closely with him or her to provide services to the population of people registered with that practice. Such 'GP attachment' has the advantages that:

• The professionals only need to liaise with a few GPs – sometimes only one practice – making communication quicker and more effective.
• All that or those practices' patients are seen by the same small district nurse team or health visitor(s).
• The attached professionals can work more closely with the rest of the practice team, facilitating, for example, the use of shared protocols for treatment.

There are, however, some disadvantages to attachment: the practice area (that is, the area within which people are allowed to register with a practice) can be very large, and there may be more scattered 'outliers' beyond that. Professionals may therefore travel longer distances to visit patients on their caseload than they would if they worked in a geographical patch. This both takes more time from that available for patient care, and costs their employing trust more in mileage allowances for staff. Attachment of staff can also lead to a situation in which a number of different district nurses or health visitors are calling on households in the same street, because their patients are registered with different surgeries. This can be perceived as illogical and wasteful by the public. However, the emphasis on teamwork and GP practice-centred primary care (see Chapters 3 and 4) will probably ensure that practice attachment continues to be the norm for these staff.

THE PRACTICE-BASED TEAM

This team – the inner core in Figure 2.1 – usually consists of attached district nurses and health visitors, and GP-employed practice nurses.

The development of some of the common nursing roles in primary care, and an overview of their roles, will be briefly reviewed before the topic of teamworking in the primary health care team is explored in the next chapter.

DISTRICT NURSING

District nursing, sometimes called 'Nursing in the Home', has existed since the beginning of the century. William Rathbone is credited with instituting a system of visiting of the sick in their homes by nurses in Liverpool in the nineteenth century. District nurses were employed by local authorities until the reorganization of the health services in 1974, when the responsibility for community nursing was transferred to health authorities. With the inclusion of community nursing services in the GP fundholding scheme in 1993, district nursing became a part of the service which was subject to contracts between GP fundholders or health authority purchasers, and the community Trusts who employ them.

The role of the district nurse is to manage and deliver nursing care to people in their own homes, and other similar settings such as residential homes and day centres, and to promote health in the broadest sense. For this role, district nurses require a number of different areas of competence:

• Technical nursing skills, which are increasing in scope and complexity with the early discharge of patients from hospital, the increasing range of treatments and equipment used to deliver them, and the trend to enable patients to choose where they wish to be cared for, allowing very ill patients with complex needs to remain in their own homes.

• Case management skills: the district nurse carries out assessment of patients' needs in the context of their home and family, designs a care plan to meet those needs, contributes to the implementation of the necessary care and coordinates the input from other professionals and services, and evaluates the outcomes of care until the patient can be discharged from the caseload.

• Staff/team management skills: many district nursing services are organized into teams, consisting of qualified and unqualified staff with different levels of skills. The district nurse 'team leader' coordinates the work, training and appropriate deployment of other members of the team.

• Liaison and facilitation: with the increasing overlap between health and social care, district nurses work alongside other services such as social services, private care organizations and voluntary organizations in the care of their clients. In addition, there has been an increasing emphasis on the primary health care team as a whole in recent years (see next chapter), so district nurses frequently need to coordinate their work with that of other professionals in primary care.

Although a district nurse qualification is not a prerequisite for working in the community (there are staff nurse posts in the district nursing team), courses have existed for several decades. Originally shorter courses of approximately 12 weeks, district nurse courses now exist at diploma and degree level. Community Health Care Nurse (CHCN) courses at degree level provide a majority of shared modules with other community nurses, and some specialist district nursing modules, leading to the award of a BSc in Community Nursing.

HEALTH VISITING

Health visiting, or public health nursing, has its origins towards the end of the last century when 'women sanitary inspectors' were employed by the public health departments of London boroughs, originally to inspect the premises where women worked and to correct poor conditions such as overcrowding and lack of ventilation. Public health work remained the focus of the profession for some years, though in 1890 the Manchester and Salford Ladies' Health Society employed women 'visitors', generally credited with being the first health visitors, partly from concern about the infant mortality rate. By the beginning of the twentieth century, more health visitors were employed specifically to extend the work of infant welfare centres into the home. As with district nurses, it was not until 1974 that health visitors were employed by the health services rather than local authorities, and in 1993 the health-visiting service became subject to contract between purchasers and providers.

The role of the health visitor is built on four principles, formally identified by the Council for the Education and Training of Health Visitors (CETHV) in 1977. They are:

- the search for health needs
- the stimulation of the awareness of health needs
- the influence on policies affecting health
- the facilitation of health-enhancing activities.

The activities necessary to put these principles into practice have also been described by the CETHV. They are:

- identifying and fulfilling health needs
- providing a generalist 'health agent' service to individuals and communities
- monitoring health needs and demands of individuals and communities, and both contributing to their fulfilment and facilitating care by other professional groups.

In practice, these activities often include child and family health monitoring, health promotion activities with all age groups, child protection work and work with community groups. An important part of the health visitor's role, sometimes claimed to be unique to the specialism, is public health activities. These often include work to reach vulnerable people who may not be reached by the rest of the primary care team: for example, because they are not registered with a GP. Homeless people, new immigrants to the country, people who travel as a lifestyle and people who live in hostels are examples of groups whose health needs may not be identified or addressed through the GP practice-based system.

To undertake all aspects of their role, health visitors work in a variety of settings: homes, health centres, child health clinics, hostels and community group settings such as church halls and community centres.

Like district nurses, health visitors work as part of the primary health care team, and need to coordinate their activities with those of other members of the team. Child health work, for example, may be shared with the practice nurse who undertakes child immunization, and health promotion activities cannot be undertaken in isolation from other, surgery-based health promotion work.

Health visitors' work is also concerned with social circumstances as well as health status, since both affect the health needs of families. They need to liaise closely with social, housing and other services, in order to help clients address their health needs. Child protection work, in particular, calls for close liaison and cooperation between health and social services, the police, the education services and others.

Unlike district nurses, health visitors rarely work in teams with a mix of skills and grades, although some work with health care support workers. Instead each health visitor assumes responsibility for a caseload of families, and works independently of other health visitor colleagues with those families. In addition, a percentage of health visitors' time is spent on public health activities: that is, activities aimed at whole communities rather than focused on individual families. To fulfil all these aspects of their role, the skills required of health visitors can be summarized as:

- technical skills, such as child health developmental assessment and group work skills
- case management skills, which involve assessing and prioritizing needs and demands from families on the caseload, and balancing family with public health work
- liaison and coordination skills, acting across the interfaces with social and other services
- health needs assessment skills, including 'profiling' the caseload and the geographical area, and identifying 'hidden' health needs in vulnerable populations
- political and advocacy skills, to bring unmet needs and public health needs to the attention of relevant authorities.

The health visitor qualification is the only community nurse qualification which is statutory (a prerequisite to employment as a health visitor) and registrable with the United Kingdom Central Council for Nursing, Midwifery and Health Visiting (UKCC). Courses leading to the health visitor qualification have been based in higher education since the 1960s, and are currently at degree level. Like district nurses undertaking the BSc in Community Nursing, health visitors share many modules with other community colleagues before undertaking specialist health-visiting modules, to become Community Health Care Nurses (CHCNs).

PRACTICE NURSING

The direct employment of nurses by GPs began many years ago, but was comparatively rare before the 1966 Charter for the Family Doctor Service, which gave GPs considerable financial assistance to employ staff. At this time, practice nurses worked principally as treatment room nurses, undertaking traditional nursing tasks, such as changing dressings and giving injections, under the direction of the doctor.

The 1990 GP Contract (see Chapter 4), however, gave practice nursing its biggest impetus, and contributed to a trebling of practice nurse numbers, to around 20,000 (9500 whole time equivalents). The Contract gave GPs financial incentives to perform screening and preventive tasks, such as taking cervical smears and immunizing children. In addition, the Contract offered similar incentives to carry out programmes of health promotion, and chronic disease management for conditions such as diabetes and asthma. In order to offer such services in addition to meeting increasing demand for traditional consultations, many practices employed practice nurses for the first time, and many others increased their practice nursing hours.

As a result of these developments in general practice, the role of the practice nurse now encompasses both the traditional treatment room tasks, including treatment of minor and chronic wounds, and the more recently acquired work of health promotion, screening, prevention and chronic disease management. In this arena, practice nurses have developed asthma and diabetic clinics, they provide travel health advice and immunizations, they undertake cervical smear programmes, and set up patient groups for education about aspects of health, or support for health-enhancing activities such as losing weight or stopping smoking.

Practice nurses are based in the GP's surgery, but also work in other settings. They may visit patients' homes, or other domestic settings such as nursing or residential homes, in order to carry out preventive work such as immunizations, and screening work such as health checks on elderly people, which are a requirement of GPs' terms of service.

One of the characteristics of practice nursing is that the nurse has an ongoing relationship with patients, who are registered with the practice, and therefore may be in intermittent contact with the nurse over a period of many years. This long-term contact facilitates the building of a relationship of trust based on an often intimate and holistic knowledge of the individual in the context of their family, work and social environment. An additional feature of practice nursing is the registered patients' ease of direct access to the nurse. Most surgeries allow patients to make direct appointments with the nurse, so that many consultations with the practice nurse are initiated by patients who attend without a prior diagnosis, or instructions from the doctor. The practice nurse is required to assess both the patient and the presenting problem, and his or her own professional competency to deal with it. For this reason practice nurses often work to surgery protocols which set out the circumstances and the extent to which they can treat a particular condition, and when referral to the GP or another professional colleague is indicated.

The skills required in practice nursing can be summarized as:

- technical skills such as venepuncture (taking blood samples), ear syringing, immunization and wound dressing
- health promotion skills, which include helping individuals to take action to improve or protect their health, as well as

running groups to educate and support people with health or information needs

- patient management skills, including assessment and appropriate referral as well as prioritizing and planning treatment
- chronic-disease-monitoring skills, which include patient education, technical skills, and a deeper understanding of the natural history of certain chronic conditions and their treatment
- programme management skills: organizing clinics, arranging for the call and recall of patients as necessary, and targeting patients for health promotion, screening and preventive activities.

There is currently no prerequisite qualification for nurses entering practice nursing. Short courses (some only 5 days in length) on practice nursing for those already in post have largely been supplanted by more substantial courses at diploma level. Practice nursing is also a branch of the Community Health Care Nurse course, in which shared community nursing modules and specialized practice nursing modules lead to a BSc in Community Nursing. Most practice nurses also attend short courses based on clinical topics such as diabetes or women's health in order to keep up to date with developments in treatment and care. Longer, more specialized courses, such as the Asthma Diploma, allow individual practice nurses to obtain specific skills relevant to their practice.

COMMUNITY MENTAL HEALTH NURSING

This community specialism started with the employment in the 1950s and 1960s of 'outpatient nurses' by psychiatric hospitals. Their role was to visit ex-patients at home, monitor their medication and offer ongoing support. When, in 1971, the Seebohm Report on social services led to the integration of the former mental welfare officers into generic social work teams, the gap in community mental health provision began to be filled by the setting up of community psychiatric nurse teams.

By 1990 there were around five thousand community psychiatric nurse posts: the ratio of CPNs to population of a district varying around the country.

> ⚠ **A Mental Health Nursing Review in 1994 recommended that all nurses working with people with mental illness should be known as mental health nurses, whether hospital or community based.**

In many areas, mental health nurses working in primary care are still known as community psychiatric nurses.

Mental health nurses working in primary care may be based in health centres or community mental health centres, and take referrals from both GPs and psychiatrists. Some are regarded as part of primary health care teams, while others are part of a mental health team. They may specialize in dealing with a particular client group, such as children and adolescents, or specialize in a particular form of intervention such as family therapy.

Educational preparation for this role takes place at pre-registration, when, following the Common Foundation Programme, nursing students follow the mental health branch of the nursing diploma. There is also a community mental health option in the CHCN degree level course.

COMMUNITY MENTAL HANDICAP NURSING

> **!** In recent years, the term 'learning disability' has largely replaced 'mental handicap', and it is the term used by the UKCC to describe this area of specialist practice in community nursing.

Nursing people with learning disabilities in the community is a relatively recent trend. This area of nursing was first described in the early 1980s, and mirrors the trend towards enabling people who would once have been confined to institutional care to live in more domestic settings and become part of a local community. Learning disabilities nurses work in multidisciplinary teams which include social workers, occupational therapists, speech therapists and others. The setting for their work may be a group home or flat, housing people with learning disabilities, a day care centre or adult training centre.

The principal areas of work in this area of nursing include:

• assessment of an individual's potential
• helping the individual to achieve his/her potential, through behaviour modification, occupational or play therapy
• managing challenging or aggressive behaviour
• integrating the individual into the community
• supporting carers and families.

Educational preparation for this area is as described above for mental health nurses. Post-registration, the CHCN course includes specialist modules for nurses working with people with learning disabilities.

COMMUNITY CHILDREN'S NURSING

The employment of qualified children's nurses in the community began in the 1950s, and developed in response to government reports emphasizing the importance of keeping children in their own homes for treatment whenever possible. Compared with other community nurses, their numbers are small, with the RCN Paediatric Community Nurses Forum putting their numbers at 120 in 1994.

The role of community children's nurses is to provide nursing care, support, information and resources to sick children and their families in settings outside of acute hospitals. A vital part of the delivery of these elements of the role is the need to sustain and nurture the relationship between the child and its parents or other carers. Community children's nurses also act as an information and teaching resource for other community nurses.

Having qualified children's nurses working in the community allows children needing complex, specialized treatment, monitoring or care to be maintained at home, and allows them to be discharged earlier from hospital when they have been admitted. In order to provide this service, a number of different schemes around the country have been set up using different models:

• A specialist community children's nurse may work as an individual in a multidisciplinary primary health care team.
• Teams of community children's nurses have been set up in some areas where there is large demand – for example, in inner cities.
• In 'inreach' schemes, community-based children's nurses maintain some responsibility for and contact with children during short periods of hospital admission
• In 'outreach' schemes, hospital-based paediatric nurses provide technical support to children in their own homes when complex treatments or equipment are in use.
• Some community children's nurses are highly specialized, focusing solely on particular conditions such as cystic fibrosis, diabetes, asthma or cancer.

The qualification of Registered Sick Children's Nurse has existed since a separate register was created for it in 1919. More recently, the nursing diploma course undertaken by pre-registration students has included a child branch following the Common Foundation Programme, allowing students to qualify for this part of the Register.

SCHOOL NURSING

School nurses' work was described in the Court Report in 1978. Elements of the role included:

- representing health in the everyday life of the school
- providing health surveillance of school children
- acting as first point of contact on health service matters
- maintaining contact with teachers over health and family problems of individual children
- teaching and offering health counselling to children.

School health services vary in size and organization in different parts of the country. Some school nurses have responsibility for many schools, others for only one or two. Their focus on school populations rather than geographical or GP-registered populations makes it more difficult for them to integrate fully with primary health care teams (PHCTs). However, some of them work in joint initiatives with members of PHCTs, such as health visitors or practice nurses, where there is a common element to their roles. Common examples are in providing contraceptive and sexual health services to teenagers, and in monitoring childhood asthma.

Post-registration school nursing courses have in the past been relatively short – lasting only weeks – and unidisciplinary. However, school nursing modules are now available in the CHCN degree course, shared with other community colleagues.

DEVELOPING ROLES IN PRIMARY CARE

The increasing emphasis on a 'primary care led NHS' has led to the development of new roles in nursing in primary care, as well as major changes to the workload of nurses in existing roles. One such new role is that of the 'nurse practitioner'. Originating in the USA in response to the shortage of medical practitioners in primary care, the role of the nurse practitioner in the United Kingdom is the subject of some controversy. The term is used to refer to nurses with a range of skills, working in different ways and having undertaken different educational preparation. In broad terms, however, the nurse practitioner is differentiated by:

- additional knowledge and skills-based training (including, for example, knowledge of pharmacology and skills such as advanced physical assessment)
- a greater degree of autonomy (usually characterised as accepting 'undifferentiated' patients, that is, patients who have not already been diagnosed by a doctor).

Nurse practitioners are usually directly employed by GPs, but some are employed by Trusts, particularly to work with vulnerable groups such as the homeless.

THE DEVELOPING PRIMARY HEALTH CARE TEAM

The roles described above are those of only some of the many different professionals working in primary care. Some of these practitioners would define themselves as part of the primary health care team, others might argue that they are part of different teams, while others, whose roles are not described here, would claim to be developing their role and moving into PHCTs in some areas. Examples of these are dietitians, physiotherapists, retail pharmacists, counsellors and complementary therapists. It is clear that there are no firm boundaries to such teams: increasingly, primary health care services are open to change and development in both their personnel and the scope of the service offered.

The Primary Care Act 1997 opened the way for more fundamental changes to the way that primary care is organized and provided: some of the pilot projects made possible by the Act have nurses providing most primary care services, and employing GPs to provide medical services.

SUMMARY

The range of different areas of nursing in primary care, the differences in their preparation, and the different focus for their work, illustrate the way that primary care has developed over the course of this century:

• The development of health visiting to encompass both public health and family health reflects the change from a collective to an individual focus in health and social welfare matters (although a public health perspective is now re-emerging: see Chapter 12).
• The development of practice nursing reflects the increased emphasis on the GP list as the focus for primary care, and on health promotion and prevention activities in general practice.
• The development of specialisms in children's nursing and care of people with learning disabilities is a consequence of the recognition of the needs and rights of these vulnerable groups in society.
• The advent of very specialized roles reflects the increasing technological and clinical complexity of treatments and equipment available to treat these conditions.

Separate and varied preparation for these different roles has been replaced by a recognition of the common skills and experience required with the introduction of the Community Health Care Nurse course.

But some differences still remain between the nursing members of primary health care teams:

• Some are employed by GPs, some by Trusts.
• Some of these are employed by community Trusts, some by mental health and some by acute Trusts.
• Some define their client group by geographical area, some by registration with a GP, some by the school attended, some by a clinical condition or disease.

The way in which these different elements of nursing in primary care work together in primary health care teams is explored in the next chapter.

Further reading

Littlewood J, ed. 1995 Current issues in community nursing–primary health care in practice. Churchill Livingstone, Edinburgh

Gastrell P, Edwards J, eds. 1996 Community health nursing–frameworks for practice. Baillière Tindall, London

Smith J. 1896–1996: a history in health. The Health Visitors' Association, London

3

Teamworking in primary care

There are references to 'primary health care teams' (PHCTs) in many NHS policy documents on primary care, and reports on nursing in primary care, as well as in textbooks and other literature. These references assume firstly the existence of such teams, and, secondly, that their constituents work together as a team, rather than acting solely as individuals. This chapter looks at the different characteristics of teams, how PHCTs fit with these models, and how teamworking in primary health care has been encouraged and supported.

DEFINING A TEAM

 A team is usually defined as a group working together to achieve a common aim.

The success of teamwork often depends on a number of factors about the team itself. These include:

- team cohesion: how the team is brought together and operates together
- its structure
- its motivation
- its self-awareness.

Variations in the *cohesion* of teams are illustrated by the differences between teams which are brought together involuntarily, as in a team of workers, with an element of chance; and those in which the members are voluntarily linked by a common enthusiasm and skill, such as a football team.

The *structural* basis of the team: the extent to which team members share common practical characteristics, such as employer, method of working, level of autonomy, and payment.

The *motivation* of such sporting teams is usually competitive, pitting members against other teams, while teams of rescuers at a disaster, for example, work collaboratively.

There are variations in the *self-awareness* of the team: in some teams the members are all explicitly aware of, and involved in forming, the joint goals of the team – sporting teams are the most obvious example – while others, such as the staff of a hotel, may only articulate a general goal: 'we are here to look after the guests'. These four dimensions of teamwork can be represented graphically, and applied to different kinds of teams (see Figure 3.1) while remembering that no combination of the four characteristics is 'correct', or necessarily better than another.

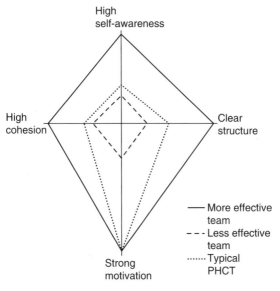

High
self-awareness

High
cohesion

Clear
structure

——— More effective team
- - - Less effective team
······ Typical PHCT

Strong
motivation

Fig 3.1 Dimensions of team characteristics.

PRIMARY HEALTH CARE TEAMS

As described in Chapter 2, there are many variations on the individuals who could be included in the primary health care team. Generally, however, the term PHCT is taken to mean the GP and the practice-based team (practice nurses and, sometimes, managers and others) together with the attached nurses from the 'community', such as district nurses and health visitors. This team is defined by the fact that they provide primary care to patients registered with one or more GP practices. Other professionals, who define their client group by other means (e.g. school nurses, or patch-based midwives), may still regard themselves, and be regarded by others, as part of a primary health care team. This is often referred to by the term 'the extended PHCT' or the 'wider' PHCT, as opposed to the 'core' (practice population-based) team.

The identification of the team is further complicated by the fact that most of the constituents of any PHCT will also be members of other teams. A district nurse will be part of a district nursing team as well as of the PHCT based in a practice. Some staff will also be attached to more than one

GP practice if one of the practices has a small list size. They then have to function in more than one PHCT as well as in a team defined by specialism.

Applying the dimensions of team characteristics illustrated in Figure 3.1 to a typical core PHCT, the following situation could be expected:

• Cohesion: the way in which the team is brought together and operates together – a typical PHCT is brought together by combining the attached district nurses and health visitors of a practice with the staff employed directly by the GP(s): that is, practice nurses, practice managers and other staff. There is an element of chance therefore, in the composition of the team: the attached staff do not apply to become members of that particular PHCT, and the GP does not generally choose the individual trust-employed staff that will be attached to his/her practice.

• Structure: the fact that there are different employers for different members of the team (Trust and GP), and therefore different management and employment practices, can weaken the sense of cohesion in the team.

• Motivation: although at a basic level the PHCT share a common objective – to care for patients, promote health and prevent ill health – there may be less agreement about methods and priorities. Trust-employed nurses may have priorities determined by trust policies or the terms of their contracts with purchasers, while GPs and their employed staff work to a different, nationally set GP contract (see Chapter 4). At times these different motivators may appear to lead the team in different directions, or by different routes to the same goal.

• Self-awareness: there have been a lot of initiatives in recent years to promote primary health care teamworking, some of which are described below. Teams which have participated in these initiatives, or read some of the literature surrounding them, may be more aware of their team roles, factors which help and hinder their teamworking, and some of the tools used to aid self-awareness and diagnose team weaknesses. Other teams may have been encouraged to reflect on their functioning with the advent of new ways of working such as the creation of integrated teams and generic team leaders (see Chapter 8).

In general, PHCTs have a number of inherent difficulties to overcome if they are to work well. An Audit Commission report summarized the situation as follows.

'Separate lines of control, different payment systems leading to suspicion over motives, diverse objectives, professional barriers and perceived inequalitites in status, all play a part in limiting the potential of multiprofessional, multi-agency teamwork. For those working under such circumstances, efficient teamwork remains an elusive ideal' (Audit Commission 1992).

However, there are also a number of factors which predispose to successful working in the primary health care team:

• Team members work with the same population of patients or clients (even if they work with different individuals).
• They often share premises.
• They all work within primary care.
• They have complementary skills, and refer clients to one another as necessary.
• There is now a shared educational preparation for community nurses.

TEAMWORK

Numerous writers have listed the essential ingredients of successful teamwork, and there is a considerable degree of agreement between them. Two examples are Firth-Cozens (1992) and the Harding Report (DHSS, 1981). Firth-Cozens identified four key characteristics of a successful team:

• having a common goal
• having a diversity of skills and knowledge
• mutual support for team members
• effective management of conflict.

The Harding Report similarly listed:

• a common objective for the team
• clear understanding by each team member of their role, function and responsibilities
• a clear understanding by each team member of the role, function, skills and responsibilities of each other team member
• a mutual respect allied to a flexible approach.

THE PHCT AS A TEAM

One of the chief characteristics of the PHCT is that is consists of a range of different professionals. They share a common objective in terms of their global commitment to restoring, protecting and promoting the health of the patient, but they may differ in the actions or the methods they use to achieve that aim.

Apart from the differences between medicine and nursing, which have to be overcome if the PHCT is to work together successfully, there are also historical and entrenched differences between the subdivisions of community nursing. The reasons for these have been listed as:

- Each subdivision was brought in for a different purpose.
- They have been established for different lengths of time.
- Each has its own culture, philosophy and representative body.
- They are managed in different structures.
- They have different educational backgrounds.
- They work with different sections of the population.
- They work in different settings.
- They have developed different skills.
- They practise at different levels (from individuals to communities).
- They work to different goals with different people (Cain et al 1995).

These origins were explored in more detail in Chapter 2.

Given these marked differences and divisions between the community nursing groups, it would be surprising if individual team members started out with a clear understanding of each other's roles. This is one of the factors often addressed in teambuilding initiatives, or informally by team members in team meetings.

The need for mutual respect and support, common to all teams, is perhaps even stronger in a team with as many inherent difficulties as the primary health care team. This too is often explicitly addressed in teambuilding events.

TEAMBUILDING INITIATIVES IN PRIMARY CARE

One of the best known teambuilding initiatives is the Health Education Authority's teambuilding workshop programme (Lambert et al 1991). This was set up in 1987, and consisted of a series of facilitated workshops, usually lasting two or three days, with overnight stays in between, for a small number of primary health care teams. Each team attending a workshop brought a number of representatives (GP, district nurse, health visitor, practice nurse, practice manager, administrative staff, for example). The goal of the programme was to promote health and reduce ill health, but other aims included the stimulation of better communication and teamwork, and the development of mutual support networks within PHCTs. This model was used all over the country, with many PHCTs finding the opportunity to take 'time out' from work to plan and socialize together as a team very valuable.

However, some teams found it impossible to take two days away from their work commitments, and others were not convinced of the benefit of explicit teambuilding activities. Other models for developing teamwork have been explored: these include team approaches to health needs assessment and practice profiling, which have the improvement of team cohesion and effective working as implicit rather than explicit aims. Another common development is the 'integrated nursing team', which will be described in more detail in Chapter 8. This is partly a practical management tool, allowing community and practice nurses to combine their skills under one team leader, but it is also used to overcome the differences arising from their different employment situations and consequent different lines of accountability, so acting as a teambuilding initiative as well.

SUMMARY

The factors which make teams and teamwork successful have been established. Although they have many positive features, PHCTs are disadvantaged in respect of some of these factors, and various explicit teambuilding initiatives have been developed to try to remedy this situation.

References

Audit Commission 1992 Homeward bound: a new course community health. HMSO, London

Cain P, Hyde V, Hawkins E, eds 1995 Community nursing–dimensions and dilemmas. Arnold, London

DHSS 1981 The primary health care team: Report of a Joint Working Group of the Standing Medical Advisory Committee and the Standing Nursing and Midwifery Advisory Committee (The Harding Report). HMSO, London

Firth-Cozens J 1992 Building teams for effective audit. Quality in Health Care 1:252–255

Lambert D, Spratley J, Killoran A 1991 Primary health care team workshop manual: a guide to planning and managing workshops for PHCTs. Health Education Authority, London

Further reading

Gillow J 1996 Team building in primary health care teams. In: Gastrell P, Edwards J (eds) Community health nursing–frameworks for practice. Baillière Tindall, London

Anon 1991 Primary health care team workshop manual: a guide to planning and managing workshops for PHCTs. Health Education Authority, London

4

General practice

INTRODUCTION

General practice is probably the most familiar setting for health care in the UK:

- 95 per cent of the British population are registered with a general medical practitioner (GP).
- 80 per cent of registered patients visit their GP at least once in a year (Fry et al 1995).
- Only 14 per cent of the population will be admitted to hospital in a year, so general practice is for most people their principal form of contact with the NHS.
- There are 30,000 GPs in the UK.

A series of Government White Papers, Acts of Parliament and policy statements, from the late 1980s to the Primary Care Act 1997 and the White Paper 'The New NHS', has made it clear that the care of people in contact with the primary health care services is structured around the general medical practice. The introduction of fundholding, making GPs purchasers of care for their registered patients, was only one clear example of this policy in practice. The current pilot schemes of 'locality commissioning', which give groups of GPs decision-making influence over the health services purchased for the patients in their area, is another. The new Primary Care Groups, to be set up from April 1999, will be led by GPs, with community nurses represented on their governing bodies. All of these schemes give GPs the power to decide, amongst other commissioning decisions, the quantity and scope of community nursing services which will be available for their patients.

In the past, in some areas, this has led to changes in the way these nursing services are structured and delivered. In others it has led to attempts to dispense with parts of the service. So it is impossible to consider any aspect of community nursing, in the present or the future, without also understanding and considering the role of general practice. This chapter reviews the history and development of general medical practice in the UK, the recent major changes which followed the 1990 reforms, and some key facts about the way in which general practice operates.

HISTORY OF GENERAL PRACTICE

ORIGINS

The origins of British general practice can be found several centuries ago with the development of three kinds of doctor (see Box 4.1).

> **Box 4.1** The origins of the general practitioner
>
> 'Physicians' in the seventeenth and eighteenth centuries were members of a learned profession. 'Surgeons' were craftsmen, and these two specialties had Royal Colleges dating from the seventeenth century. The 1815 Apothecaries Act created the Society of Apothecaries: 'apothecary-surgeons' were generalists who undertook care of people in the community. These 'general practitioners' had developed from both the physician and surgeon branches of the profession, with the strongest link being with the surgeons; hence GPs' premises and consultations are still referred to as 'surgeries' today (Loudon 1986).

In 1858, the Medical Registration Act imposed some structure on the profession of medicine, aiming to end what has been described as 'the evils of rampant quackery and illegal practice. The absence of uniformity in training or examination. The jealousies, antipathies and hostilities between the members of the profession' (Rivington 1989). It also formalized the system of referral letters from a GP to a consultant which still exists today. In this way 'the physician and surgeon retained the hospital while the GP retained the patient.' (Stevens 1966).

> ⚠ **The need for a patient to have a referral letter from his or her GP to gain access to the hospital services is the basis of GPs' claims to have the 'gatekeeping' role in the NHS.**

DEVELOPMENT

During the Industrial Revolution, in the 1850s, Sick Clubs were formed in the poorer areas as small, prepaid insurance schemes for workers and their dependents. The National Health Insurance Act of 1911 allowed all workers below a certain wage level to 'register' with an approved GP, who received 'capitation' payments (that is, a payment per head) to provide what were called 'general medical services'. Under this scheme, families and dependents were not covered, and had to pay fees for services.

The 1946 National Insurance Act extended this insurance to everyone of working age, except some of the non-employed. It included married women, who were covered by their husband's contributions.

By 1948 the National Health insurance scheme covered half the population; the other half included children, self-employed people and many old people. Access to suitable services also varied depending on location. As much of GPs' earnings still came from private patients, GPs were concentrated in more affluent areas.

THE NATIONAL HEALTH SERVICE

The National Health Service Act of 1946, which set up the National Health Service in 1948, extended the established national health insurance principles to the whole population. This meant that everyone could register with a GP of their choice, who would receive capitation and other fees to provide all general medical services, including referral to NHS specialists when necessary.

GPs were fiercely resistant to the setting up of the National Health Service, and mass resignations were threatened. One of the most significant aspects of the National Health Service Act was that it did not, in the end, make GPs employees of the new service. Alone amongst doctors, GPs retained independent contractor status. They worked – and continue to work – to a nationally negotiated contract with the Department of Health, providing their services to their registered populations in return for capitation fees, and other fees and allowances.

THE GENERAL PRACTITIONERS' CONTRACT

ADMINISTERING THE GPs' CONTRACT

When the health service was first set up, the GPs' contract with the (then) Ministry of Health was administered by Executive Councils, replacing the former insurance committees. The Executive Councils evolved through reorganizations over the years into Family Practitioner Committees (FPCs), then Family Health Services Authorities (FHSAs), before the FHSAs and District Health Authorities were replaced by new Health Authorities following the Health Authorities Act 1995.

GENERAL PRACTICE TODAY

> ⚠ **The independent contractor status of GPs is one of the most important characteristics of this part of the health service, affecting their payment, accountability, workload and organizational structure.**

The key facts about general practice shown in Box 4.2 all arise from the fact that they are independent contractors rather than employees of the health service.

Box 4.2 Key facts about GPs and general practice

• GPs do not receive a salary, but instead claim a series of fees and allowances for aspects of their work (see Box 4.3).
• The total amount which would be earned by an average GP providing the normal range of services is recommended each year by the Doctors' and Dentists' Pay Review Body, and any changes made to the amount of each fee reflect this 'average' remuneration.
• GPs do not have 'managers': managers within FPCs, FHSAs and now Health Authorities administer the GP's national contract on a day-to-day basis, dealing with claims for fees and ensuring that GPs meet their 'terms of service' under the contract, but they do not have managerial authority over GPs.
• GPs can directly employ the staff they need to help them run their practice: these include managers, administrative staff and nurses. These staff are not employed by the NHS, but by the GP, and until 1997, were not therefore eligible for the benefits of other NHS employees such as access to the NHS pension scheme.
• GPs in group practices work together under a legal partnership agreement – they are not co-employees of a practice organization.
• The average individual GP list size is 1865 people, although some have as many as 2500–3000 registered patients.

Box 4.3 Examples of GPs' fees and allowances

Fees:

• capitation fees per registered patient
• item of service fees for carrying out particular tasks such as adult immunizations, giving contraceptive advice, or giving maternity care
• target payments for reaching a set percentage of a target population with services such as childhood immunization or cervical cytology screening.

Allowances:

• for seniority within the practice
• for completing postgraduate education
• for working in an area of particular deprivation.

THE DEVELOPMENT OF GP CONTRACTS

In the years immediately following the creation of the NHS, GPs worked in a way that remained largely unchanged for twenty years. They provided primary medical services to patients registered with their practice, and referred those patients on to specialist, hospital-based services when necessary. However, facilities and equipment in practices were often minimal, many GPs worked without partners or staff, and their practices were often housed in very basic premises.

1965

In 1965, the Charter for the Family Doctor Service was written by the General Medical Services Committee (GMSC) of the British Medical Association (BMA). Although GPs campaigned against a new contract based on the Charter, a contract was negotiated with the Government which made significant changes in the structure of British general practice. Amongst other provisions, GPs were given financial assistance to obtain suitable premises, and to employ practice receptionists, secretaries and nurses. Following this, more group practice partnerships were formed, and more practices worked from new premises and health centres.

1990

The most recent contract between the Department of Health and general practice came into effect in 1990. For the first time, this contract set out specific objectives for general practice concerning availability to patients, preventive activity such as health promotion, the supply of information to patients and the provision of information to the (then) FHSAs for management purposes. This contract too was resisted by GPs, and its imposition was markedly unpopular.

Effect of the 1990 Contract on practice nursing The introduction of fees for health promotion work, and for reaching targets in child immunization and cervical screening, led to a rapid and eventually three-fold rise in the number of practice nurses employed by GPs. What had begun as a numerically small part of community nursing, generally undertaking treatment room duties delegated by the GP, developed into a significant and much more autonomous role as practice nurses took on and developed health promotion, immunization and screening services in general practice.

THE 1990 REFORMS

As well as the new GP contract, 1990 saw the enactment of the NHS and Community Care Act which set in motion the wide-ranging health service reforms of the 1990s. Two major and inter-related elements of the reforms particularly affected general practice: the introduction of an internal market in health care, and the introduction of GP fundholding.

THE INTERNAL MARKET

The effect of the internal market – separating the 'purchasing' of health care from the provision of health care – has been described in Chapter 1. GPs' reactions to the prospect of this change were largely negative: 'more than three-quarters of the 2231 GPs who replied [to a Medeconomics survey] felt their independent contractor status and clinical freedom would be restricted; nor did they believe that any real improvement in the management of primary care would be achieved' (Leathard 1990).

FUNDHOLDING

GP fundholding was one of the major planks of the internal market. Instead of providing general medical services to their patients, and referring them on to hospital specialists for secondary care, GPs were offered the opportunity to hold the budget for some of that secondary care. They could then make contracts with different hospitals, specifying the amount and quality of care they wanted for their patients, and choosing between a number of competing providers on the basis of both price and quality of care. If they saved any money out of their fundholding budget, it could be reinvested in the practice or used to purchase further services. The benefits of fundholding were proposed as:

- improving the quality of services on offer to patients by GPs
- helping GPs develop their practices for the benefit of patients
- allowing GPs greater control over the use of resources for their patients
- encouraging hospitals to be more responsive to the needs of GPs and their patients.

The first 'wave' of 306 fundholding GPs took on the role in April 1991, and further waves started each subsequent April until 1998, when most of the eighth wave was suspended while the new Labour Government considered the future of the internal market.

Fundholding was not originally intended to devolve to GPs the total responsibility for purchasing all the services required by their patients. However, a number of different models of fundholding developed over the life of the scheme:

- In 'standard' fundholding, fundholders purchased drugs, staffing and accommodation, community nursing and a range of elective secondary care surgery and outpatient services.
- 'Community' fundholding, introduced in 1993, excluded the secondary care surgery from the scheme.
- Pilots of 'total purchasing' allow fundholders to contract for and purchase all services for their patients if they choose to do so.
- Various forms of 'extended' fundholding allow practices to add some of the less predictable and potentially expensive elements of need, such as accident and emergency or maternity services, to their contracts.

FUNDHOLDING REVIEWED

When the fundholding scheme was reviewed in 1997/98, following the change of Government, a number of criticisms were being levelled at it.

> ⚠️ **The most serious criticism was that it created a two-tier system of health care, overturning the founding NHS principle of equity.**

Specific criticisms were:

- Fundholding GPs' patients were said to be 'fast-tracked' through hospital waiting lists so that the Trust could fulfil the terms of their contract with the GP and retain their contract in the next negotiating round.
- Fundholders' patients could sometimes be treated while other elective work was suspended because fundholders still had funding when the health authority had used all their funding prior to the end of the financial year.

Another significant criticism was that the time and cost of individual, annual, contract-setting between GP fundholders and Trusts outweighed the cost-cutting benefits of competition.

Among the benefits of fundholding, it was claimed that:

- Hospital waiting lists had been shortened.
- More attention was paid to the quality of care patients received.
- Better services could be provided in practices using fundholding savings.

Even amongst fundholding GPs, however, support for the fundholding scheme was not unanimous. A survey in 1994 identified that 15 per cent of *lead* partners in fundholding practices did not support fundholding, and a further 5 per cent classified themselves as 'don't knows'. Amongst other GP partners in fundholding practices, levels of support for the scheme were even lower, with 55 per cent saying they did not support fundholding (Appleby 1994).

In 1996, an Audit Commission report, 'What the doctor ordered', reviewed the overall impact of the fundholding scheme. It concluded that:

> 'most fundholders have mastered the considerable administrative burden, but in purchasing terms they are only maintaining the status quo. They are making changes at the margins, but continuing to purchase the same services, in the same quantity, from the same providers as the health authority purchased on their behalf before they became fundholders'.

The White Paper 'The New NHS – Modern, Dependable', published in 1997, signalled the end of fundholding, with no new admissions to the scheme, and current fundholders' participation ending in April 1999.

THE EFFECT OF FUNDHOLDING ON COMMUNITY NURSING

Purchasing services

Community nursing was one of the services purchased by fundholders under any of the different variants of the scheme. This led some fundholders to review their need for the different elements of community nursing: specifically, some questioned the need to purchase health visiting in the quantity and to the specification that they used to receive from health authority purchasers. Some fundholders used their purchasing power to try to change the focus of the service, while others chose to increase community nursing provision.

However, it was not only GP fundholders who carried out such reviews of community nursing services. Some health authority purchasers made similar changes, including large-scale cuts, to community nursing, in order to redeploy scarce financial resources elsewhere in the health service.

Managing community nurses

It was also common for GP fundholders to want to have a greater influence over the day-to-day management of community nurses, even though the nurses are still employed by a Trust. Integrated nursing teams, led by one of the community nurses acting as 'team leader' or team coordinator, were developed, allowing the whole nursing team – including GP employed practice nurses – to work more closely with a GP practice (see Chapter 8).

LOCALITY COMMISSIONING

With the review of the internal market in 1997, and the possibility of changes to fundholding, came the proposal of 'locality commissioning' as an alternative way for GPs to become involved with and influence the purchasing of services for their patients. Locality commissioning groups had existed in parallel with fundholding in some areas. They consisted of a group of GPs who met to identify the needs of their combined registered patient populations, and to advise the health authority purchaser about commissioning health care to meet those needs.

In 1997, with further interest in developing models of locality commissioning, a number of pilot areas were set up by the Department of Health to try out different ways of making locality commissioning work in a more formal way. Each locality commissioning group has either an actual budget, devolved from their local health authority, or a 'notional' budget: that is, a paper budget to work within, rather than control of the funds. All locality commissioning pilot groups have responsibility for their combined prescribing budget.

The commissioning groups have to carry out needs assessment of the population they cover – varying from around 40,000 to nearly half a million people – and commission health services necessary for that population. The GP commissioning groups have been explicitly encouraged to involve other members of the primary health care team in their work, and evaluation of these pilot schemes, due after 2 years, will show how successful they have been. The successful commissioning groups are likely to act as models for the new Primary Care Groups which will have the same commissioning remit.

GENERAL PRACTITIONERS AS EMPLOYERS OF NURSES

GPs have employed practice nurses for many years, but there was a steep rise in the numbers of nurses employed in this way following the introduction of the 1990 GP contract. These nurses are not employed by the NHS, and therefore do not have automatic right to the terms and conditions of services that NHS employment confers. The clearest example of this is that, until the Primary Care Act, 1997, practice nurses could not join the NHS pension scheme. There are a number of advantages and disadvantages to direct employment by GPs. The advantages often cited by practice nurses are:

• freedom from nurse management hierarchies

- a high level of autonomy in practice
- opportunity to negotiate directly with employer regarding grading, training and development opportunities, and changes to practice and role.

There are, however, a number of disadvantages identified by nurses who are directly employed by GPs:

- conflict that arises when demands from employer seem to oppose professional requirements
- difficulty in negotiating directly over pay and conditions
- professional isolation
- lack of locally accessible professional nursing guidance.

In spite of these difficulties, surveys have shown that practice nurses are generally more satisfied with their jobs than other nurses, and most practice nurses would not want to be employed by Trusts instead of GPs.

SUMMARY

General practice has a long history in the UK, long predating the setting up of the National Health Service. GPs have retained their 'gatekeeper' role of being the main point of referral to the rest of the NHS. GPs are not employees of the NHS, but independent contractors.

The 1990 GP contract gave them newly-formalized responsibilities for preventive and screening activities, and many practices took on practice nurses, or increased their practice nursing hours, to meet these obligations.

Fundholding allowed participating GPs to purchase community nursing services from Trusts, and gave them an interest in shaping and controlling those services. The Primary Care Groups which will be active from April 1999 will require GPs and community nurses to work together to assess the health needs of their local population and commission health services to meet those needs.

References

Appleby J 1994 Data briefing: fundholding, Health Service Journal, 11 August

Audit Commission 1993 Practices make perfect: the role of the Family Health Services Authorities. HMSO, London

Audit Commission 1996 What the doctor ordered? A study of GP fundholders in England and Wales. HMSO, London

Fry J, Light D, Rodnick J, Orton P 1995 Reviving primary care: a US–UK comparison. Radcliffe Medical Press, Oxford

Leathard A 1990 Health care provision–past, present and future. Chapman and Hall, London

Loudon I 1986 Medical care and the general practice–1750–1850. Clarendon Press, Oxford

Rivington W 1989 The medical professions (Carmichael Prize Essay). Royal College of Surgeons, London

Stevens R 1966 Medical practice in modern England; the impact of specialization and state medicine, Yale University Press, London

Further reading

Leathard A 1990 Health care provision–past, present and future. Chapman and Hall, London

Fry J, Light D, Rodnick J, Orton P 1995 Reviving primary care: a US–UK comparison. Radcliffe Medical Press, Oxford

SECTION 2

Nursing in primary care

5

Patients and clients

The terminology applied to people who use the health services in primary care settings varies depending on the setting and the professional group involved with them. Some nurses use the term 'patients', others prefer 'clients' or 'service users', or simply 'users'. However, some people find this unacceptable because of the association with drug 'users'. People in nursing homes, or group homes for people with learning disabilities, may prefer the term 'residents'. For the purposes of this chapter, the term 'patients' will be used for simplicity, while acknowledging that this may sometimes be inappropriate in practice.

For most nurses working in hospital, 'their' patients are all or some of the patients on their ward or in their department. The patients are defined by their physical presence in the nurse's place of work. In primary care, however, this is not always the case. Many community nurses work in people's homes, or in settings such as schools or workplaces, where people do not attend primarily to see the nurse. This chapter looks at the ways in which nurses and other professionals, working in different settings in primary care, acquire their patients.

WHERE PATIENTS COME FROM

There are four main ways in which people find their way into the daily work of community nurses. These are:

- by being 'registered' with a GP
- by being on a 'caseload'
- by being referred to the nurse or health visitor
- by referring themselves to an 'open access' service.

REGISTERED PATIENTS

People who are registered with a GP remain patients of that GP's practice until they register with another practice, or, rarely, are removed from the list of registered patients by the GP. Even if they never attend the surgery, or use the practice's services, they are still registered patients. Practice nurses are employed by GPs to work with the registered practice population, so all the patients on the GP's list are also patients of the practice nurse, whether or not they use the nursing services of the practice. In this way a practice nurse theoretically has a patient population of around 2000 people per GP in the practice. However, some people on the GP's list will never attend to see the practice nurse, and others will only attend occasionally, while some will return regularly for appointments with the nurse as well as the doctor.

Access to the practice nurse for patients registered with the practice is usually available by two routes: by referral from the GP, and by self-referral. The GP will refer a patient to the practice nurse for a specific intervention (such as a wound dressing, immunization or blood test), or for longer-term management of a chronic condition requiring education, monitoring, support and treatment review (such as diabetes, asthma or coronary heart disease).

Patients self-refer to the practice nurse for a range of investigations, treatments, and screening and preventive activities which are carried out with reference to a practice protocol rather than on direct instructions from the GP. The advantages to patients of being registered with a practice, and so having a practice nurse available, are:

• They become familiar with one nurse, or a small team of nurses, over a period of time.
• They have direct, local access to nursing advice and expertise without having to be referred by a doctor.

Patients will remain with their practice nurse as long as they are registered with the same GP practice.

CASELOADS

People may become part of a caseload by virtue of a 'universal' system, or a 'targeted' system. The traditional health visitor's caseload of under 5 year olds is an example of a universal system. The community nursing services are notified of all babies' births in their area, and every family with a new baby becomes part of the caseload of a named health visitor. Usually this is the health visitor 'attached' to the GP practice with which the baby's mother is registered. In some areas of the country this process takes place during the mother's pregnancy, allowing the health visitor to make an antenatal visit to the family. Other areas are moving away from universal health visiting, arguing that, after an initial visit, some families do not need to remain on an active caseload, but can be left to call on the health-visiting service when they have a specific need. Families or individuals with particular needs or at particular risk can then become part of a 'targeted' caseload. In the case of health visitors, caseloads are not confined to families with young children. Patients may become part of a health visitor's targeted caseload because of bereavement, age (some health visitors work with older people) or because they request such support. Other examples of universal caseloads are those of the school nurse, who is responsible for the health needs of the population of one or more schools, and the occupational health nurse, who fulfils the same function for employees of a particular firm. The advantages to patients of being on a caseload are twofold:

- They have a named person whom they can contact for advice or support.
- The caseload holder has a responsibility to actively assess the health needs of the individual or family, rather than waiting to be called upon.

Patients will remain on a caseload until either they reach a cut-off point defined by age – for example, a child starts school and moves from the caseload of a health visitor onto the caseload of the school nurse – or they no longer require the service.

REFERRAL SYSTEMS

Patients may become part of community nurses' workload by means of referral from a GP, another nurse, another health professional, or another source. District nurses' patients are often referred to their service by their GP. Where district nurses are attached to a GP practice, their referrals will come from the GPs in that practice. If the district nursing team is patch-based, then they may take referrals from many different GP practices, depending on where the residents of their patch are registered. The GP referral may be for a specific nursing intervention such as wound dressing, or for assessment where the patient's condition is giving cause for concern. The district nurse 'caseload holder' will then assess the patient, and devise a plan of care, in conjunction with the patient and family, which may be implemented and evaluated by different members of the district nursing team. When the patient is assessed as no longer in need of nursing intervention, he or she will be discharged from the service.

Community mental health nurses, community paediatric nurses and Macmillan nurses work in a similar way, receiving referrals from GPs and others, but because they are fewer in number, they are more likely to receive referrals from a number of practices.

GPs are not the only source of referrals to community nurses. Interprofessional referrals, either nurse to nurse, or other professional to nurse, are becoming more common. One of the major advantages of teamwork between different professionals and groups in primary care is that it makes it easier for patients to receive the range of care and expertise they need. Rather than the patient having to return to their GP time and time again to be referred for different treatments or advice, one member of the team can act as coordinator of care, with other members of the team making and receiving referrals as appropriate throughout the course of the patient's illness or time of need (see Figure 5.1). The advantages to the patient of referral systems are:

- A professional or other qualified/experienced person can

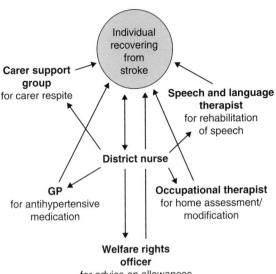

Fig 5.1 An example of interprofessional referrals.

judge which service is the most appropriate to refer to, and when is the most appropriate time to refer.
• They allow patients access to a range of services and professionals which do not accept self-referrals by patients.

OPEN-ACCESS SERVICES

These are services which do accept direct contacts from patients. Common examples within the health service are:

• district continence advisory services
• diabetes and other specialist nurses' services
• 'well woman' or contraceptive services
• clinics or services for homeless people or drug users.

Private nursing services to which the public have direct access include:

• nursing and home care agencies
• occupational health nurses (who have a direct-access service for the employees of a company)
• nurses in private schools.

In some areas, services such as health visiting have an open-access element in addition to the caseload element. For example, an individual may request a visit from a health visitor when he/she has a particular need, such as bereavement or family problems. Open-access services are frequently advertised through posters and leaflets in public places and GPs' surgeries, through publicity on local radio 'health slots' or at health fairs, and by talks to pre-existing groups such as playgroups or women's groups. In order to meet diverse and unpredictable levels of demand, these services need to be flexible and responsive, offering a choice of times, venues and services. The advantages to the patient of open-access services are:

• They do not need to identify their need to a third party in order to ask for referral.
• They can choose the time, place and type of service which they feel is most appropriate to them.

Generally, contact with an open-access service lasts as long as the patient chooses to make use of the service.

SUMMARY

Patients can make use of the community nursing services in primary care by being registered with a GP, being part of a universal caseload, or being referred to a service. They can also choose to access some services directly. This multiplicity of approaches can cause confusion to people who are not familiar with the health service. It is sensible not to assume that people know how to contact nursing services, and to explain the different mechanisms if there is any possibility that an individual may need them, or that they may not understand why a particular service has been offered to them.

6

Settings for care

Primary care has already been loosely defined as care taking place in settings outside acute hospitals. By this definition there are many different settings for nursing in primary care. The only thing such settings have in common is how different they are from the acute hospital setting. They differ in:

- size
- formality
- how well-equipped and resourced they are
- level of hygiene
- level of safety.

Some places where nursing care is provided by community nurses are:

- patient's homes
- GPs' surgeries and health centres
- residential homes and warden-controlled flats
- drop-in centres
- informal settings, e.g. the streets.

Each of these places has different implications for practice.

NURSING IN PATIENTS' HOMES

District nurses carry out most of their clinical work in the patient's home. Health visitors, clinical nurse specialists (in continence or diabetes, for example) and Macmillan nurses will also visit people at home. Other community nurses, such as practice nurses, will also do some home visiting for patients who cannot attend the GP's surgery.

 The most important thing to remember about working in a patient's home is that you are only there with their permission.

Nurses do not have a right of entry to the home, and if you outstay your welcome, or act in a way that is unacceptable to the patient, you may be asked to leave, and not allowed to return. Not only is this difficult for you, but it could cause the patient to refuse entry to other health professionals in future, leading to the individual or family missing out on essential care or treatment in the future. To minimize the chance of any problems when working in patients' homes, remember:

- Leave gates as you find them.
- Use doorbell if available and working, rather than banging on doors.

- Allow plenty of time for people to answer the door, especially if elderly or disabled.
- Always show your identification and allow people time to check it.
- Always introduce yourself by name.
- Make sure you are dressed professionally, whether in uniform or your own clothes.
- Be courteous to everyone in the house, not just the patient.
- Be careful not to cause damage to furniture by carelessness with liquids or sharp instruments.
- Remove clinical waste and sharps, following Trust or surgery procedures, and ask permission before disposing of other waste in the household bins.
- Respect patients' cultural traditions concerning their homes, families and contact with outsiders.

Once in the patient's home, the equipment and space available for carrying out treatment, or taking measurements of the patient's vital signs, may not be ideal. The level of cleanliness, quietness, privacy and time available will vary from home to home.

> ⚠ It is important to adapt procedures to the informal setting, while maintaining the important principles (see Box 6.1).

Box 6.1 Adapting a principle of care to different settings

Principle – prevention of infection

Examples of application:

- Use cleansing hand rubs rather than hand washing if facilities not available.
- Screw top jars can replace conventional sharps bins if necessary.
- A clean field can be created on a settee, pavement or car seat by using a sterile paper towel.

There are many advantages to visiting patients in their own homes:

- Patients can be assessed in their everyday setting, so difficulties they might have in complying with suggested treatments or lifestyles can be spotted. *Example*: suggesting hot baths to relieve the stiffness of arthritic joints will be inappropriate if the patient does not have regular access to hot water, or cannot get into the bath.

• Patients are more relaxed, and may tell you important things about themselves or their condition which would not be revealed in a surgery consultation. *Example*: an elderly person may respond to a comment about their pleasant 'granny flat' by saying that they feel cut off from the rest of the family.

• A person in their own home is more in control of the situation, and is better able to ask for information or to explain why they do or do not want a particular treatment. *Example*: a woman may discuss with the community midwife the different options available to her during labour without feeling that there is a busy clinic of other mothers outside the door.

Disadvantages of visiting patients in their own homes are:

• It takes more time than seeing people in clinic or surgery premises, because of travelling and the need to adapt procedures to different homes.

• All equipment and resources that might be needed have to be carried to every visit.

• A car is essential for most community nursing posts, though some practitioners, particularly students, manage on public transport.

• Personal security can be a problem for nurses working alone in people's houses, and travelling between visits (see Chapter 9).

• Employers (trusts or GPs) have to pay travelling expenses incurred as part of community nurses' work.

NURSING IN GP SURGERIES AND HEALTH CENTRES

Practice nurses spend most of their time working in GP surgeries, or the health centre in which their employing GP has a practice. District nurses and health visitors often hold clinics in surgeries or health centres in addition to visiting people at home. These settings vary from large modern centres equipped to carry out some operations and investigations such as gastroscopies, to converted houses, or even pubs. When working in surgeries or health centres, remember:

• The premises belong to either the trust or the GP, so treat them with care.

• There is likely to be great demand on rooms and equipment; be considerate of other professionals, and check before using a room.

• Reception and clerical staff have to deal with the public, often under great pressure, throughout the day; treat them with respect and courtesy.

• Health and safety legislation applies to these premises; you have a duty to take reasonable care to prevent accidents and injuries, and to report any incidents that do occur.

The advantages of seeing people in a health centre or surgery are:

• More people can be seen in the time available. *Example*: in a leg ulcer clinic lasting 1 hour you could probably dress six ulcers, rather than the two or three you could see in patient's homes.
• It is easier to communicate with other professionals, both by writing in the client's notes in the surgery, and by verbal communication with other staff *Example*: if you were advising a woman about emergency contraception, and she needed an immediate prescription, you could see the GP, probably within a few minutes, to arrange this.
• The equipment and other resources you need are more likely to be at hand. *Example*: if you are teaching an asthmatic child how to use a new inhaler, the surgery or health centre probably has a range of placebo inhalers and information leaflets or videos which could help in the teaching process.
• You are usually safer from the fear or threat of violence in premises which are staffed throughout the day, and used by many people.

The disadvantages of working in these premises are:

• There are often a lot of people around, with noise, numbers and interruptions creating a more pressured feeling for the patient.
• There may be less space and privacy than would be available in a patient's home.
• People have to travel, and often wait, in order to receive treatment or advice; this may be particularly difficult for the elderly, frail or disabled, and for people with children.
• The premises may be inaccessible, or difficult to access, for people with restricted mobility.

NURSING IN RESIDENTIAL HOMES OR WARDEN-CONTROLLED FLATS

District nurses may have patients resident in these homes or flats who require their services because the Home's staff are not qualified to provide nursing care. Practice nurses also sometimes visit residential homes, to carry out immunizations against influenza, for example. Clinical nurse specialists will also visit patients who live in residential homes or flats. The important factors to remember when working in these settings are:

- The residential institution or controlled flat is the patient's home, and should be treated with appropriate respect.
- The manager or warden of the home or flats may want to be informed of your visit, possibly on every occasion, and may suggest that certain days or times of day are most convenient for your visit; check with him/her on your first visit.
- Security is important; if you enter through a communal door before going to the patient's room or flat, make sure it is closed again behind you.
- If there is an intercom or entryphone, encourage the patient to choose a codeword you can use; saying only 'it's the nurse from the surgery' makes it too easy for someone else to impersonate you and gain entry.

The advantages of nursing people in these settings are:

- They are in a familiar environment, so less prone to confusion or anxiety than might arise, for example, if they had to be admitted to hospital.
- There are other people around who may be able to help the patient, for example, to wash in spite of a cumbersome bandage or dressing.
- There are staff or a warden who can report whether the patient is coping with being cared for in this way.

The disadvantages are that your visits may have to fit in with the routine of the Home, or of the warden of the flats; and visits may take longer than usual if you liaise with the staff or Warden before or after your visit.

DROP-IN CENTRES

These can be held in health service premises, such as clinics, or other premises such as community halls, hostels or schools. Drop-in sessions sometimes provide some appointment slots which can be pre-booked, but often all or part of the session is available for people to present themselves without an appointment. Many different community nurses provide drop-in sessions, for different clients: see Table 6.1. The advantages of seeing patients in this way are:

- Patients can choose when and how often to come. *Example*: a homeless person might attend a nurse practitioner's drop-in session every week to have his sore feet dressed.
- They don't need to be referred by a doctor or other health professional. *Example*: a schoolgirl might want advice about sexuality and relationships without involving her family's GP or practice nurse.
- They can sometimes be anonymous or use a pseudonym if they want, depending on the nature of the session. *Example*: drop-in sessions are commonly held at genito-urinary

Table 6.1
Examples of drop-in clinics which may be run by nurses

Practitioner	Drop-in clinic
School nurse	Counselling General health advice Sexual health and contraception Smoking cessation
Practice nurse	Young person's health check Minor illness clinic Women's health sessions
Health visitor	Baby/child clinic Young person's advice Pre-conception clinic Women's health sessions
Nurse practitioner	Minor illness clinic General health advice and treatment

medicine (GUM) clinics, and clients have a choice of whether to give their real name, a pseudonym, or choose a reference number.

• People who are not registered with a GP, who are transient in an area or lead disorganized lives for any reason know that they can always access health care and advice at these sessions. *Example*: a drug addict might have difficulty finding a GP who will allow her to register, but could use a drop-in sexual health clinic for contraceptive advice, cervical smears and general health checks.

• For nurses running these sessions, one advantage is that they can be held in many different places, making it more likely that people in need will come to them.

• They provide the satisfaction of bringing care to people who might not have received it through more formal channels.

The disadvantages of drop-in clinics are:

• The premises may be far from ideal for delivering nursing care.

• The number of people who will attend any session is unpredictable, so it can be difficult to plan timing efficiently.

• Because people self-refer to the session, the problems they bring may be beyond the scope of the nurse running it – a list of names and contact details of people to whom patients can be referred on is essential, together with a clear understanding of professional accountability in practice (see Chapter 8).

Nurses working with homeless people, or people with substance abuse problems, sometimes carry out at least some of their work in the very informal settings where they find their clients. These may be on a park bench, in a subway or a shop doorway. Nurses also work from vans providing mobile services on the streets, or taking screening services to workplaces and schools.

These must be the most challenging settings in which nursing in primary care takes place. Even so, these settings have some advantages:

• The client does not have to make contact with the health service by, for example, trying to register with a GP (often impossible if he has no address), nor travel to an Accident and Emergency department.
• Advice and health education can be directed at the most practical and relevant aspects of the client's life, such as the essentials of nutrition.
• The client's personal and financial circumstances and lifestyle are clearly seen, so irrelevant and impractical advice is avoided.

The disadvantages, of course, are significant:

• The nurse only has access to whatever equipment, information and resources he/she can carry, or is available in the vehicle.
• Travelling time, and time spent finding and befriending clients, is considerable.
• Clean surfaces and washing facilities are often unavailable, to the nurse at the time, and to the client subsequently.
• The nurse's personal safety can sometimes feel jeopardized in these settings.

APPLYING PRINCIPLES TO DIFFERENT SETTINGS

Working in these different settings provides a range of very different experiences for community nurses. However, some general do's and don'ts apply whatever the individual client's circumstances, and whatever the setting for care.

Do:

• Apply the Code of Professional Conduct in every situation
• Know and follow Trust or surgery protocols on clinical issues such as immunization, infection control and the administration of medicines
• Follow principles rather than procedures where necessary

- respect the client's home or environment, however inadequate it seems
- be prepared to spend a lot of time for little apparent gain
- accept that small improvements are as significant as large ones
- be vigilant about personal safety and avoid unnecessary risks.

Don't:

- treat people's homes like hospital wards or clinic rooms
- treat people's homes like your own home
- expect people to conform to your procedures or timetable
- impose your values or standards on other people
- offer treatment or care regimes which are impossible to follow because of the client's lifestyle or circumstances.

SUMMARY

Nursing in primary care takes place in a wide variety of settings, all of which have both advantages and disadvantages in the provision of care. It is essential that nurses are flexible and creative in their approach to the care and treatment of people outside traditional clinical settings.

7

'Patients' in primary care

When a person is in hospital, they are, of course, usually referred to as a 'patient'. People who are registered with a GP are also generally referred to as the GP's 'patients'. However, for much of the time, people do not consider themselves to be patients in the sense of needing treatment for an illness or injury. In primary care, many of the people nurses deal with are neither ill nor injured. Their contact with the health service is simply to receive a service which relates to their health or wellbeing. Examples are:

- contraceptive services
- health promotion services
- child development checks
- immunization
- general health screening
- breast or cervical screening services.

For this reason some community nurses refer to the people they work with as clients, or residents, or simply families or individuals. This distinction is important for more than semantic reasons. It reflects two key factors which make people receiving services in primary care different from patients in hospital. These are:

- a much greater degree of choice, autonomy and control
- ongoing relationships with nurses and other professionals.

CHOICE, AUTONOMY AND CONTROL

People in the community have many more choices about their health care than people in hospital. They therefore have much greater autonomy of action, and a greater degree of control over their pathway through the health services. For example, they can choose:

- which doctor's practice (if any) they register with
- whether and when they want to see a doctor, nurse, health visitor or other professional
- whether they keep the appointment they have made
- whether or not they take a prescription to the chemist to obtain the medicines prescribed
- whether they then take the medicine, and if so, whether or not they follow the doctor's or pharmacist's instructions, how long they take it for, and whether they pass it on to someone else
- whether or not they follow other advice such as about diet or exercise
- whether and when they attend for follow-up consultations with the doctor or nurse; and, most significantly
- whether they choose to live in way which minimizes damage to their health.

There are many other examples of choices people can make, and areas of their health care over which they have control.

In contrast, a patient in hospital is visited by professionals to their timetable and at their instigation, given medicine and expected to take it to a schedule, and given the recommended diet and treatment for their condition. Even where changes towards a more patient-centred approach have been implemented, the whole ethos of the hospital inpatient experience is conformance and loss of control. Of course this is often necessary when the success of care or treatment relies on compliance with an optimum 'care pathway'. In primary care, however, health is usually not the main focus of people's lives, and the requirements of health care are susceptible to the individual's priority setting.

This situation, of choice and control by the individual, requires a very practical response from nurses in primary care. In order to work in partnership with individuals, nurses need to:

- negotiate rather than impose (appointments, treatments, offers of help or advice, access to homes)
- give information to make choices rather than give solutions
- accept that people will make choices which could be regarded as unwise or unhelpful
- be prepared to act as advocate for the individual with other professionals when they put their choices into effect.

Some individuals or groups of people may have less choice than others, because, for example, their health, lifestyle, education or language means that they cannot understand the choices available, or cannot take advantage of them. In these instances, the advocacy role of the nurse is even more important.

ONGOING RELATIONSHIPS

Unless someone is unfortunate enough to have a longstanding, serious illness, they are unlikely to have long-term relationships with nurses based in acute hospitals. In primary care, however, ongoing relationships with members of the primary health care team are much more common:

- GPs often have people registered with them for years, and get to know them through consultations for a variety of reasons; often a whole family is registered with the same practice, so all members are known to the doctor.
- Practice nurses, working for GPs, also have long-term relationships with all members of the family, not only through episodes of illness but through consultations about, for

example, contraception, travel vaccines, childhood ailments and health checks.

• Health visitors still often retain families on their caseload for the first 5 years of a child's life, and in addition can undertake long-term support of people who have suffered bereavement.

• School nurses get to know children and families through years of progression through school.

• District nurses often provide care to people with chronic, sometimes terminal illness, visiting frequently and spending significant amounts of time over a long period with the same family.

• Community mental health nurses have long-term clients whom they help to maintain in the community through supervising treatment and undertaking therapeutic support work.

The long-term nature of the relationships between nurses in primary care and the individuals with whom they work mean that:

• Interpersonal skills are very important for work in primary care.

• Holistic care, dealing with the individual in the context of family and community, has to be a reality.

• The work can be both more stressful and more rewarding.

THE PATIENT'S CHARTER

The Patient's Charter was introduced by the Department of Health in 1991, with a summary document sent to every household in the country. It was described in the foreword to the document by the then Secretary of State for Health as 'the central part of the Government's programme to improve and modernize the delivery of the service to the public, whilst continuing to reaffirm the fundamental principles of the NHS'.

The Charter contained 10 charter 'rights' for patients (see Box 7.1) and 9 national charter standards. Some of these standards concerned intangibles such as the right to respect for privacy, dignity, religious and cultural beliefs; others were specific, covering, amongst other things:

• waiting time for ambulances answering emergency calls (14 minutes in urban areas, 19 minutes in rural areas)
• time between arrival and assessment in accident and emergency departments (seen and assessed immediately)
• waiting times in outpatients' departments (seen within 30 minutes of appointment time).

District health authorities were required to publish details of their performance against these standards in five key areas,

> **Box 7.1** The 10 patient's rights contained in the Patient's Charter
>
> - to receive healthcare on the basis of clinical need
> - to be registered with a GP
> - to receive emergency medical care at any time
> - to be referred to a consultant under certain circumstances
> - to be given a clear explanation of any treatment proposed
> - to have access to health records
> - to choose whether or not to take part in medical research or training
> - to be given detailed information on local health services
> - to be guaranteed admission for virtually all treatments by a specific date no later than 2 years from the day when the consultant places the patient on a waiting list
> - to have any complaint about NHS services investigated.

and update their reports annually, as well as providing the name of the person whom the public could contact for information.

THE PATIENT'S CHARTER IN PRIMARY CARE

In 1992, the Department of Health launched the Primary Care Charter Initiative. This required Family Health Services Authorities (which administered the contracts of GPs) to put in place charters for their own work. It also required them to support GP practices or primary health care teams which chose to develop their own, voluntary charters. Both the FHSA and practice charters had to include a statement of patients' rights under general medical services (Box 7.2) and be based on the 'user's guide to primary healthcare' (Box 7.3).

> **Box 7.2** Patients' rights under general medical services
>
> - to be registered with a GP
> - to be able to change doctors easily and quickly
> - to be offered a health check on joining a doctor's list for the first time
> - to receive emergency care at any time through a GP
> - to have appropriate drugs and medicines prescribed
> - to be referred to a consultant when their GP thinks it necessary and be referred for a second opinion if they and the GP agree this is desirable

Box 7.2 *(contd)*

- from November 1 1991 to have access to their health records (subject to any limitations in law)
- to choose whether or not to take part in medical research or medical student training
- to be offered a yearly home visit and health check if 75 years old or over
- to be given detailed information about GP services through the FHSA local directory
- to receive a copy of their doctor's practice leaflet
- to receive a full and prompt reply to any complaints they make about NHS services.

Box 7.3   The 'user's guide to primary healthcare'

Help us to help you.

- Please let us know if you change your name or address.
- Please ask us questions if you are unsure of anything.
- Please ask for a night visit only when it is truly necessary.
- Please do everything you can to keep appointments.
- We want to improve services and will therefore welcome any comments you have.

In addition to these two elements, practice charters were encouraged to set standards in three other key areas:

- access to healthcare (for urgent and non-urgent consultation, and repeat prescriptions)
- contacting the services (how to reach a doctor or nurse by telephone in normal hours and in emergencies)
- comments and complaints (name of the person who will record and coordinate action on complaints).

The Patient's Charter (which is due to be replaced in 1998/1999 with a new 'NHS charter') is often cited as one cause of the increasing demand for primary care services, and so blamed for the general increase in workload on general practices and their teams. However, it seems likely that the general increase in consumerism in society as a whole also contributes to increased expectations of the health service. The fact that people in primary care enjoy a greater degree of autonomy and choice about their healthcare means that they may be able to pursue their 'rights' more vigorously than the relatively constrained patient in hospital.

Some people in the community are not only consumers of the health service: they also contribute to the development and monitoring of services. This can take a variety of forms. The commonest are:

- patient participation groups
- neighbourhood forums
- community health councils
- the Patient's Association.

Patient participation groups are usually based in a GP practice. People who are registered with the practice either volunteer for or are co-opted onto a group which represents the views of the users of the practice services. Some of these groups are very active, discussing with the practice staff representatives all practice developments, such as improvements to premises or changes to appointment systems. Others have a more marginal role, which may focus on raising money to buy extra clinical equipment or additional items for the public areas of the premises.

Neighbourhood forums have a wider membership, often including representatives from the police, social services, local churches, schools and youth workers, as well as health services representatives and residents. They discuss both social and health issues, and sometimes lead the way on joint projects which will improve local people's lives as well as having an impact on their health, and their need for health services.

Community Health Councils were set up as statutory bodies in each health district in 1974. Their remit is to represent the interests and views of the consumer of health services, and to monitor the services. Although financed by the then Area Health Authorities, they were intended to be independent bodies, with half their members nominated by local authorities, some by regional health authorities and others by voluntary agencies. There are 211 CHCs in England and Wales, recommending improvements to local health authorities based on the views of their communities. Their meetings are open to the public.

The Patients Association was founded in 1963 as a campaigning organization. It acts as an advisory service and a 'voice' for patients, independent of the Government and the health professions. It is financed by members' subscriptions, donations and a Government grant. The Association published its own 12 point patient's charter in 1991.

SUMMARY

People in the community, receiving health-related services through primary care, have a greater degree of choice and control about their health care than patients in hospital. This has practical implications for nurses in primary care, who need to work in partnership with individuals and families to help them make choices about their health, their lifestyles and the treatment options available when they are ill. The long-term relationships between the professional and the individual necessitate good interpersonal skills and a genuine commitment to holistic care.

8

Professional issues

The professional guidance and regulations which apply to registered nurses, midwives and health visitors cover those professionals regardless of where they work. Clearly they apply equally to all nurses in primary care, across the range of different nursing and related specialisms, and in the numerous settings for care (see Table 8.1).

Working in primary care, however, does have some features which make familiarity with the professional guidance even more important:

• Nurses often carry out their work in physical isolation from other nurses or other professionals (e.g. district nurses working alone in people's homes).
• They can have a high degree of autonomy in the performance of their role (e.g. deciding how to treat a wound and when to discharge a client from a caseload).
• They work with some of the most vulnerable people in society (e.g. homeless people, young children, dependent older people).
• Some are managed by non-nursing professionals or non-professionals (e.g. practice nurses, occupational health nurses).
• Many work outside the NHS (e.g. nurses in residential and nursing homes, occupational health nurses, nurses in private schools and practice nurses) and are subject to widely varying conditions of employment, training opportunities and resources for practice.

Table 8.1
Examples of nursing specialisms, settings and employers

Specialism	Setting for care	Employer
Practice nursing	General practice, homes	GP
District nursing Health visiting Community mental health nursing Midwifery	Homes, clinics, residential homes, hostels etc.	NHS trust, acute, community, combined
Nursing in private nursing homes	Nursing home	Home owner
Occupational health nursing	Employment premises	Company

> ⚠ It is essential that every nurse is able to apply the professional guidance to practice in very practical ways, and is sufficiently confident of her/his position to defend it when necessary against pressures to do otherwise.

The position statements, codes and other documents which are published by the United Kingdom Central Council for Nursing, Midwifery and Health Visiting are widely circulated to registered nurses, and available from all nursing libraries, or direct from the Council. They will be not be reproduced in detail here.

UKCC GUIDANCE

THE CODE OF PROFESSIONAL CONDUCT

The main requirements of the United Kingdom Central Council (UKCC) Code of Professional Conduct are shown in Box 8.1.

> **Box 8.1** The UKCC Code of Professional Conduct (UKCC 1992a)
>
> *Principal requirements*: Each registered nurse, midwife and health visitor shall act, at all times, in such a manner as to:
>
> - safeguard and promote the interests of individual patients and clients
> - serve the interests of society
> - justify public trust and confidence
> - uphold and enhance the good standing and reputation of the professions.

> ⚠ Registered nurses who are employed in the personal social services and residential care sector, even if their posts do not require nursing qualifications, remain subject to the Code of Professional Conduct.

THE SCOPE OF PROFESSIONAL PRACTICE

While all nurses are very familiar with the requirements of the Code of Professional Conduct, the Scope of Professional Practice position statement, published for the first time in 1992, may be less familiar. This guidance makes important changes to the way in which nurses take on new areas of practice, and is particularly relevant in primary care, where new developments (see below) have brought many new opportunities for nurses.

The term 'scope of professional practice' refers to the tasks and responsibilities undertaken by the registered nurse for which he or she is adequately trained and competent to perform. They should be related to the individual's personal experience, education and skill. Prior to 1992, nursing practice beyond the level and range of activities covered by pre-registration education – such as venepuncture and intravenous drug administration – required certification.

> **⚠ The 'Scope of Professional Practice' document ended the requirement for certificates of competence in these additional activities.**

Instead of certificates, the practitioner is required to apply a set of 'principles for practice' in deciding whether to extend their role into a new area (see Box 8.2). In effect, individual nurses decide when they are competent to take on new tasks or roles, and accept professional accountability for the new areas of work. Difficulties can arise if nurses are pressured by employers to take on new areas of work when they do not consider themselves to be competent.

Box 8.2 The principles for adjusting the scope of practice (UKCC 1992b)

'The registered nurse, midwife or health visitor:

- must be satisfied that each aspect of practice is directed to meeting the needs and serving the interests of the patient or client
- must endeavour always to achieve, maintain and develop knowledge, skill and competence to respond to those needs and interests
- must honestly acknowledge any limits of personal knowledge and skill and take steps to remedy any relevant deficits in order effectively to meet the needs of patients and clients

Box 8.2 *(contd)*

- must ensure that any enlargements or adjustment of the scope of personal professional practice must be achieved without compromising or fragmenting existing aspects of professional practice and care
- must recognize and honour the personal accountability borne for all aspects of professional practice
- must, in serving the interests of patients and clients and the wider interests of society, avoid any inappropriate delegation to others which compromises those interests.'

 If there is no local source of professional advice and support, contact the representative of your professional association for advice in these circumstances.

POST-REGISTRATION EDUCATION AND PRACTICE

The aim of the UKCC's Post-Registration Education and Practice (PREP) programme is to develop individual nurses, midwives and health visitors in order to maintain and improve standards of patient and client care.

 For midwives, the current system of statutory refresher courses continues to be valid until superseded by the full PREP requirements in April 2001.

The four key elements to PREP, which will enable practitioners to renew their registration when it becomes due, are:

- completion of a notification to practice form
- a minimum of 5 days or equivalent of study activity every 3 years
- maintenance of a personal professional profile containing details of professional development
- a return-to-practice programme if the individual has not practised for a minimum of 750 hours or 100 working days in the 5 years leading up to renewal of registration.

'Study activities' can include attending seminars, distance learning, visits to other areas of practice or personal research, as well as attending a course. Combining some of these methods makes it possible for nurses who work part-time, or who have difficulty acquiring study leave from their employer, to fulfil the study requirements.

There are five key categories in which study can be undertaken:

- patient, client and colleague support
- care enhancement
- practice development
- reducing risk
- education development.

OTHER UKCC GUIDANCE

Separate guidance exists on confidentiality, accountability, the administration of medicines, records and record keeping, complaints about professional conduct and clinical supervision. Each of these contains:

- principles which must be applied to practice in all settings
- some specific guidance for work in community settings, patients' homes and non-NHS settings.

> ⚠ **All nurses in primary care should have access to copies of these documents, and be familiar with their content.**

PROTOCOLS AND GUIDELINES IN PRIMARY CARE

One of the consequences of the physical isolation of community nurses is that they frequently work at a distance from other members of the team. This makes standardization of a service, and consistency of practice, more difficult than it would be if professionals could observe each other's practice. Partly in an attempt to address this, protocols or guidelines are often produced for all members of the team to use. In addition to ensuring consistency between professionals, they can ensure that identified best practice is followed, and individual variations are minimized.

The term 'protocols' is usually used to mean a check list of items which are to be undertaken. A protocol for an immunization clinic, for example, will cover tasks to be performed, information to be given to patients, the staff to be involved and the circumstances under which patients will be referred to the doctor or have their immunization deferred.

'Guidelines' are usually less prescriptive than this, and professionals can choose to deviate from them if there is a valid clinical or professional reason for doing so.

Ideally, protocols and guidelines should be:

- agreed by all the professionals who will be using them
- based on objective evidence of effectiveness
- regularly reviewed and amended as necessary
- easily accessible to everyone who needs to use them.

In practice, protocols and guidelines are often inherited or adopted from elsewhere; this can be entirely satisfactory provided they are regularly reviewed for relevance and acceptability to the current professionals using them.

 Remember: using a protocol or guideline does not remove your individual accountability for your practice.

HEALTH CARE ASSISTANTS

District nurses, health visitors and nurses working in residential care homes or nursing homes may have health care assistants as part of their team. There is sometimes confusion about the roles and responsibilities of members of the team under theses circumstances, but the UKCC makes it clear that:

- Health care assistants to registered nurses, midwives and health visitors must work under the direction and supervision of those registered practitioners.
- The registered practitioner remains accountable for assessment, planning and standards of care, and for determining the activity of his/her support staff.
- Health care assistants should be integral members of the team.

CLINICAL SUPERVISION

Clinical supervision is a broad term which is used to cover a variety of forms of reflective practice in nursing and midwifery. It has been defined as 'the process whereby a practitioner reviews with another person her ongoing clinical work and relevant aspects of her reactions to it' (Minot and Adamski 1989).

In primary care, a range of different models of clinical supervision have been piloted, and in some cases incorporated into everyday practice (see Box 8.3). The development of clinical supervision in community nursing started with mostly unprofessional groups – groups of health visitors within a trust, or groups of practice nurses within general practice, for example – although there are a growing number of clinical supervision programmes which are set up for multi-professional, and even multi-agency, teams.

The opportunity to share concerns and achievements in practice, in the context of a safe, clearly bounded meeting or group, can be particularly valuable to community nurses. Working in isolation, making frequent, major decisions without easy recourse to colleagues, and dealing with the rapid changes in service structure which have been so common in recent years, can all put great stress on the individual practitioner. Clinical supervision provides essential support and guidance for all practitioners, not only those new to practice.

Box 8.3 Models of clinical supervision in primary care

Groups:
- unidisciplinary groups
- multidisciplinary groups
- peer-led groups
- supervisor-led groups

One to one:
- with supervisor
- with peer
- with manager

Supervisors:
- peers
- volunteers
- rotating
- higher grades
- team leaders/managers
- other professions

Activities in supervision sessions:
- significant event analysis
- case review
- topic discussion
- free discussion

! Some practitioners, who have specialist aspects such as child protection in their role, have specialized clinical supervision for this aspect of their work provided by a supervisor with appropriate clinical experience.

Where clinical supervision programmes do not currently exist, it is possible for an individual practitioner to start the process of setting them up. The King's Fund have produced guidelines on setting up clinical supervision, which are shown in Box 8.4.

> **Box 8.4** King's Fund guidelines for setting up clinical supervision (Kohner 1994)
>
> 1. Discuss and define the purpose of supervision.
> 2. Involve all staff in the planning process.
> 3. Consider qualifications, skills and experience required of supervisors.
> 4. Provide opportunities for training for all supervisors.
> 5. Arrange supervision for supervisors.
> 6. Make supervision available to all practitioners regardless of seniority.
> 7. Clearly define the content of supervision.
> 8. Formally define the relationship between supervisor and supervisee.
> 9. Plan monitoring and evaluation of supervision.
> 10. Ensure the support of the employing authority for clinical supervision.

DEVELOPMENTS IN CARE AFFECTING NURSING IN PRIMARY CARE

There have been many changes to the scope and delivery of health care, and the structure of the health services, in recent years. Some of the more significant have been:

- shorter hospital stays – discharging people 'quicker and sicker'
- new drugs and other treatments – prolonging life and allowing people to live at home with chronic diseases
- increased emphasis on consumer choice about the place and type of health care – raising expectations about control and participation
- the development of a 'mixed economy' of provision – including private-sector hospitals and nursing homes as providers of mainstream nursing and medical care.

Many of these developments have had very practical impacts on nurses in primary care. For example, they have increased the dependency of district nurses' patients, brought primary health care teams into closer contact with the personal care services run by social services departments, and enabled midwives to re-emphasize their role, in partnership with mothers, in the management of normal pregnancies.

OTHER DEVELOPMENTS AFFECTING NURSING

The political and managerial initiatives which have brought about some of these changes have also brought in a number of new terms for the different methods of service delivery. It is useful to have some understanding of these, as they are frequently encountered in primary care.

Collaborative care planning is a process in which representatives of all the professionals who will be involved in caring for people with a particular condition come together to plan a 'pathway of care' for them. The plan includes both acute (hospital) and community elements of care, and the professionals agree standards for the care to be delivered. The aim of collaborative care planning is to ensure that all patients receive the same high standard of care, to the same broad 'specification'.

Integrated care pathways, or managed care, also refers to the production of an agreed package for the care needed by individuals with a particular condition, which is intended to be consistent and seamless across primary and secondary care sectors.

A care programme approach (CPA), usually in mental health, involves the designation of a 'key worker' who coordinates a package of care for an individual client following assessment. The key worker is responsible for maintaining contact with the individual, continuously assessing need and evaluating the care delivered, and altering the plan of care as appropriate.

Integrated nursing teams are those in which all the different specialisms in nursing – district nurses, health visitors, practice nurses, community mental health nurses – work as one team. Sometimes this is accomplished by having all professionals, including practice nurses, employed by the same Trust. In other examples, the practice nurse may continue to be employed by the GP, but work as part of the integrated team. A team leader, or team coordinator, is often appointed, and may be any of the individuals within the team, or an additional post.

Hospital at Home schemes aim to provide the level and intensity of support to people in their own homes that would be available to them in hospital. By using specialist nurses (such as Macmillan nurses, or community children's nurses), additional equipment and home adaptations, it is possible to nurse people in their own homes with a range of very serious conditions, and to maintain therapies such as intravenous infusions, central lines and continuous oxygen therapy. This sort of care may prevent people having to go into hospital at all, or enable them to be discharged very early.

Intermediate care is another innovation which provides a level of care greater than that ordinarily provided by the primary health care team. Care is provided in the client's home, by multidisciplinary professionals, in order to enable people to be discharged earlier from hospital once they are medically fit, but still requiring paramedical treatment or support. It is usually time-limited, providing support for a designated period only, and so not suitable for people with long-term care needs.

PCAPs (Primary Care Act Pilots) projects are around 90 projects which are using the provisions of the 1997 Primary Care Act to try out new ways of working in primary care. Some of these pilots are led by nurses, and involve a group of nurses employing a GP on a sessional basis to provide personal medical services to a population, while the nurses provide other services. Others involve a nurse becoming a partner in a GP practice, while the GP-focused projects allow GPs to be salaried rather than independent contractors.

PRIMARY CARE GROUPS

One of the most significant developments affecting the role of nurses in primary care results from the Government White Paper 'The New NHS – Modern, Dependable'. This paper introduces a series of changes to the health service, many of which are focused on primary care. The major changes contained in the White Paper are:

- the abolition of the 'internal market'
- the ending of the GP fundholding scheme
- the requirement for all health and local authority bodies, including primary care groups, to work to an agreed health improvement programme
- the setting up of 'primary care groups', consisting of representative GPs and community nurses, together with social services representatives, to plan and commission health care for local populations.

These primary care groups will exist in all areas and represent all GP practices, and will therefore affect every community nurse. Some nurses will become representatives of their colleagues on the group, and participate in commissioning services from Trusts. Others may be involved in the profiling and needs assessment exercises which will be necessary to inform commissioning activities (see Chapter 34). Other functions of the primary care groups to which community nurses in all settings may be expected to contribute include:

- promoting the health of the local population
- monitoring the performance of Trusts against service agreements
- developing primary care through joint working, sharing skills, audit and quality review
- working with social services on the planning and delivery of services.

PUBLIC HEALTH INITIATIVES

In recent years there has been a renewed emphasis on public health, as well as individual health. Public health includes action on all aspects of people's lives which affect their health, including their environment, social and financial status, employment and housing. The contribution which can be made by every nurse, working in every setting, to public health work, is set out in 'Making it happen', a report from the Standing Nursing and Midwifery Advisory Committee (1995).

The report explains the key characteristics of a public health approach, and the contribution that nurses, midwives and health visitors can make. The key concepts underlying the work of these professions which are relevant to public health are described as:

- a 'public health' approach – involving the identification of health needs and desired outcomes, and agreement on the most effective and acceptable action and evaluation
- knowledge of population health needs even when caring for individuals
- emphasis on collective and collaborative action
- recognition of people as members of groups as well as individuals
- a public health perspective, anchoring clinical and non-clinical care in the social, organizational and policy aspects of health development
- a focus on health promotion, enabling people to increase control over and improve their health, combined with preventing disease.

Nurses can make a significant contribution to public health work, the Report argues, because:

- They are the largest professional workforce.
- They deliver a variety of services, and have a diversity of skills.
- They are in regular and close contact with clients and families.
- They see clients in their social context.
- They have privileged access to critical information about personal health.
- They have opportunities to communicate with local people.
- They are valued by society, and expected to act as patient advocates.
- They network with a wide spectrum of operational staff in statutory and voluntary organizations.

Public health is also the subject of a Government Green Paper, 'Our healthier nation', published in 1998. This sets out four priority areas for public health action, adapting those targeted through the previous Government's White Paper 'The health of the nation'. The four areas are:

- heart disease and stroke
- accidents
- cancer
- mental health.

Targets for improving health in these four areas are set out in the paper (see Table 8.2). The 'settings for action' in which preventive work will take place on these four target areas are particularly relevant to community nurses. They are:

- schools (focusing on children)
- workplaces (focusing on adults)
- neighbourhoods (focusing on older people).

'Our healthier nation' is explicit in recognizing the need for action on social, financial and other factors, as well as those directly connected with health care: 'This means tackling inequality which stems from poverty, poor housing, pollution, low educational standards, joblessness and low pay'.

> **!** Nurses in primary care are in an ideal position to identify where these factors are affecting people's health and wellbeing, and to direct any available help to tackle them.

Table 8.2 'Our healthier nation' targets	
Area for action	Targets (by 2010)
Heart disease and stroke	Reduce the death rate from heart disease and stroke and related illnesses in people under 65 by at least a further third
Accidents	Reduce accidents by at least one fifth
Cancer	Reduce the death rate from cancer in people under 65 by at least a further fifth
Mental health	Reduce the death rate from suicide and undetermined injury by at least a further sixth

SUMMARY

While all professional guidance for nurses, midwives and health visitors applies to nurses wherever they work, the particular employment arrangements and working conditions of nurses in primary care makes the application of guidance to practice a very practical activity. Nurses are ideally placed and skilled to contribute to public health work as well as work with individuals.

Developments in health care, and changes to the structural arrangements of the NHS, have introduced new terminology and ways of working to primary care. The involvement of community nurses in the new primary care groups, which have responsibility for needs assessment, health promotion and service commissioning, opens up new areas of development of nurses in primary care.

References

Department of Health 1997 The new NHS–modern, dependable. The Stationary Office, London

Kohner N 1994 Clinical supervision in practice. King's Fund Centre, London

Minot S R, Adamski T J 1989 Elements of effective clinical supervision. Perspectives in Psychiatric Care 25 (2): 22–26

Secretary of State for Health 1998 Our healthier nation: a contract for health. The Stationery Office, London

Standing Nursing and Midwifery Advisory Committee 1995 Making it happen: the contribution of nurses, health visitors and midwives to public health. HMSO, London

UKCC 1992a The code of professional conduct. UKCC, London

UKCC 1992b The scope of professional practice. UKCC, London

Further reading

Swain G 1995 Clinical supervision: the principles and process. Health Visitors' Association

UKCC 1997 PREP and you. UKCC, London

9

Mobility, safety and appearance

While many of the principles of nursing in primary care are similar to those used in nursing in acute settings, the practical issues are very different. This chapter will look at some of the most significant issues for nurses working outside of hospitals: mobility, including use of the car for work, and personal safety.

MOBILITY

Nurses working in primary care may travel about a great deal – if they carry out all their work in individual's homes – or less frequently, if they work in several health centres, or are usually surgery-based with the occasional home visit. While the use of a car is often the easiest solution to getting about in primary care, it is not the only one. In some towns and cities, public transport is so well developed, and parking so difficult and expensive, that it is easier to make use of public transport than use a car.

PUBLIC TRANSPORT

When using buses, trams and local trains, remember:

• Obtain an up-to-date timetable, as routes and services can change.
• Ask about discount tickets which save money and hassle.
• Make sure you have plenty of change if you are paying as you go.
• Carry the number of a taxi firm for emergencies or urgent calls.

 Remember the need for confidentiality: do not read or write patient notes in public places.

If you are using public transport in the course of work, you should be able to reclaim the costs of journeys from your employer. Trusts will have a public transport expenses claim form, usually completed monthly. Check with them about their policy for reimbursing taxi fares before trying to claim these. Nurses working for general practitioners, nursing homes or other private employers should negotiate reimbursement of travel expenses as part of their conditions of employment.

USING YOUR OWN CAR

Many community nurses use their own car to travel in the course of their work. Travel expenses are reimbursed at one of two levels:

• Regular car user – if the car is used a lot for work-related travel: a monthly lump is payable for wear and tear, together with an amount per mile for distance travelled in the course of business.
• Standard car user – if the car is not used so often: no monthly sum is paid, but the rate per mile is higher.

These schemes are run by Trusts, and nurses employed by a Trust should check with the expenses section of the Finance Department, or through their manager, for details of the qualifying mileage and rates of reimbursement. Nurses working for private employers will find that arrangements and rates vary considerably between employers, and they should ask for written details at the time of employment.

> ⚠ It is essential that you tell your motor insurance company that you are using your car for travel in the course of your work, and have your policy amended accordingly.

LEASE CARS

Some Trusts have a lease car scheme under which community staff pay a monthly sum, deducted from their salary, for the sole use of a car which is owned by the lease company. These cars used to be referred to as 'Crown cars'.

The advantages of this scheme are:

• The staff member can usually choose from a range of different makes and models of car.
• The cars are usually renewed every three years.
• They are covered by a motoring organization for accident and breakdown.
• The costs of insurance, road tax and routine servicing are all included in the monthly sum paid.
• A courtesy car is usually supplied during servicing or when the car is unavailable due to accident damage.

The disadvantages of this scheme are:

• The lessee never owns the car.
• The car has to be returned if the lessee leaves the job.
• The rate per mile for business mileage is relatively low.

• There are restrictions on the amount of private mileage which can be undertaken.
• The lease car is taxed as a benefit.

> ⚠ **As there is usually an excess sum to pay on the insurance, having a lease car does not solve the problem of vandalism often anticipated by community staff.**

LOOKING AFTER A CAR

Working in the community may take staff into areas with high crime rates, or entail leaving their car unattended and out of your sight for periods of the day. As damage to or loss of a car is inconvenient and disruptive to work, as well as distressing to the individual, it is worth remembering a few general precautions:

• Always leave the car locked, even if you only expect to be away a few minutes.
• Leave windows closed, however hot the weather.
• Use a simple steering wheel immobilizer as a visible deterrent.
• Don't leave a medical-type bag, nursing books or magazines, dressings or equipment on display, as these may suggest to people that you might also carry drugs, needles or syringes.
• Don't leave valuables where they can be seen.
• Don't display 'Nurse on Call' type stickers unless you are sure the supposed benefits (leniency from traffic wardens) outweigh the risks of inviting a search for drugs etc.

Some general safety precautions which apply to all motorists are shown in Box 9.1.

PARKING

Parking a car can be a problem in many residential areas, even for the residents. It is more difficult for community nurses who do not know the area and the usual arrangements. Neighbours, delivery vans and refuse lorries have been known to block in strange cars while they go about their lengthy business. To avoid problems in street parking:

• Ask the advice of colleagues who have visited the area or the street before.
• Ask the advice of the patient or client as you go into the house.

> **Box 9.1** Safety tips for motorists
>
> Community nurses' work can take them through busy city streets, or through remote country lanes; each can have its hazards. When driving the car:
>
> • Don't have a medical-type bag or handbag on the front seat beside you.
> • Don't leave a mobile phone on the seat beside you.
> • Find out your route before starting a journey, or have local street maps with you, so that you don't need to leave your car to ask for directions.
> • Keep doors locked while driving.
> • Keep change for a public telephone, and for parking, in the car but not in view.
> • Keep water, rugs or blankets, and spare petrol in the car at all times.
> • In winter, carry a shovel, boots and extra blankets in the car.
> • Let people know where you are going and when you should be back.

• Don't park in areas marked 'residents' parking': they are often rigorously patrolled.
• Don't park on the client's drive unless invited to do so.
• Don't risk parking illegally, even for a brief time.
• Don't rely on a 'Nurse Visiting' sticker to save you from traffic wardens, parking fines, or acts of aggression.

Parking in health centres is usually not such a problem, although they are often crowded and can be the scene of minor bumps and shunts. If you have to park very close to another car, or even double park other staff, leave with reception staff your name, description of your car and where you will be working, so that you can be asked to move the car if necessary.

GPs' surgeries often have limited parking, and it is frequently marked with areas for 'doctors' and 'patients'. When visiting a surgery for the first time, check with reception staff where you should park, to avoid giving cause for complaint.

PERSONAL SAFETY

Protecting personal safety requires attention to three areas:

• health and safety generally
• avoiding violence and aggression from clients
• avoiding other safety hazards.

HEALTH AND SAFETY

The Health and Safety at Work Act, 1974, requires employers to safeguard, as far as reasonably practicable, the health, safety and welfare of the people who work for them. The NHS (Amendment) Act which came into effect in 1987 lifted Crown immunity from the NHS, so that NHS employers could be prosecuted if premises or practices did not meet health and safety standards on inspection by the Health and Safety Executive.

The obligations on employers under the Health and Safety at Work Act include:

- drawing up a safety policy detailing measures to be taken to protect health and safety of employees
- identifying key individuals with relevant responsibility for health and safety
- ensuring that there is adequate provision for first aid for employees should they become ill or be injured at work.

As nurses in primary care work in a variety of premises, ranging from institutions, health centres and surgeries to village halls, people's homes and informal settings, it is particularly important that they are aware of health and safety in each location:

- Nurses working for Trusts should be able to see a copy of the health and safety policy, and be told the name of their health and safety representative. Nurses working for private employers should discuss these issues with their manager.
- The location of the first aid kit, and the name of the designated first aider should be known in case of accident or injury.
- The accident book should be easily accessible for reporting of injuries.

The Health and Safety at Work Act also places a responsibility on employees to take reasonable care to avoid injury to themselves and to others by their work activities. Employees must also cooperate with employers in meeting statutory requirements, including reporting hazards and accidents.

> ⚠ When starting a new job or placement, ask about health and safety policies, and accident reporting, if it is not included in your induction.

AVOIDING VIOLENCE AND AGGRESSION IN PRIMARY CARE PREMISES

Nurses in primary care are often thought to be at greater risk of violence and aggression than those who work in hospitals, although surveys do not always bear out this assumption. In spite of the climate of fear incited by media reports, it is worth remembering that the vast majority of patients and clients will never be violent or aggressive. However, in order to fulfil the statutory requirement to take reasonable care, and to reduce the risk of even occasional threatening incidents, there are a number of factors which can be addressed by community nurses. In relation to primary care premises, these include:

- structural factors
- procedures
- training
- use of technology
- planning.

Structural factors include the use of space and building design to reduce the risk of threats or violence to staff. There are two different schools of thought about design for safety. Some designs use glass screens and high counters to protect staff from clients. The alternative view is that such barriers increase tension, and design should be open to foster a more relaxed atmosphere. These are factors over which community nurses do not have control. The use of the existing building design, however, can be altered to reduce the risk of unmanageable situations between staff and clients. For example, if seeing clients in health centres or surgeries:

- Try to use rooms off main corridors or near reception areas rather than upstairs or at a distance.
- Arrange the seating so that the client is not between you and the door.
- Do not leave instruments on visible display which could be used as weapons.

Simple procedures which can reduce threat to staff include:

- not making appointments when there are no support staff in the building
- checking on each other if appointments seem to be taking too long
- arranging a code word or action if help is required
- giving people information about reasons for delays, treatments offered or withheld, or systems in use, to reduce their frustration and tension and prevent escalation into aggression.

Training in interpersonal skills and the management of aggression can be a very useful tool. Even simple actions, such as adopting non-confrontational postures and speaking quietly, can defuse a potentially difficult situation. If training is to be arranged, it is useful for the whole team, including reception staff, clerical staff and GPs, to take part. This helps to promote a consistent approach across all workers in the practice, as well as preventing any individual feeling that they are alone in feeling frightened or vulnerable.

Aids and technology can help to reduce risk to staff, although they can also have the effect of promoting a climate of defensiveness, or even complacency.

• Key pads on doors leading to some areas of the building can prevent unauthorized people entering.
• Bars on windows reduce the risk of intruders' entry.
• High counters and hatches protect reception areas from clients.
• 'Panic buttons' in consultation rooms allow practitioners to summon help if needed.

> ⚠️ **If any of these measures are in place, a new member of staff or student on placement will be expected to use them, whatever their personal views, as they form part of the employer's health and safety policy.**

PLANNING

The safety measures in place, and level of training and awareness amongst staff, vary greatly between areas. Often they are based on the particular practice's or team's experience of aggression, and may have developed in an ad hoc way in response to specific concerns or incidents. A better response would be a planned approach to avoiding aggression. This would involve:

• a full team discussion of their experiences, concerns and ideas
• a comparison of different methods of enhancing staff safety, and discussion of the pros and cons of each
• prioritization of the most effective methods
• implementation with training as necessary
• audit of incidents, staff perceptions and patient/client perceptions after an agreed interval prior to review.

AVOIDING VIOLENCE AND AGGRESSION OFF PRIMARY CARE PREMISES

Community nurses often feel most at risk of aggression when in people's homes, when travelling, or in informal settings such as hostels or clubs. A few well-publicized tragedies have highlighted the danger that nurses and other health workers can face. Such incidents are of course very rare. There are measures which can be taken, however, to reduce the risk of such incidents, and of more minor but still unpleasant experiences.

Structural measures include:

• noting exits and door opening mechanisms as you enter
• placing yourself nearer to the door than is the patient or client
• avoiding seeing clients upstairs if it is not necessary because of their physical state.

Procedural measures include:

• checking the address and name of the client with other members of the team to see if there is a history of problems
• taking a colleague with you on a visit if there is reason for concern
• keeping a daily diary at a central point, such as a health centre or manager's office, so that people know where you are and when you are due at another visit or back in the office.

Training in handling difficult situations has already been discussed. It is important that any such training for staff who will be travelling and visiting alone includes this aspect of work, as well as dealing with situations where there are other staff on shared premises.

Aids and technology are often considered the mainstay of security for nurses who travel and make house calls. Mobile phones or two way radios are undoubtedly useful, but it is important to remember that you may not have an opportunity to use them in a situation of threatened violence. Attack alarms can disorient temporarily, and may draw attention to an emergency situation, but they will not necessarily bring help. As with every other measure, they have to be part of a planned and considered strategy for increasing safety, rather than the whole answer.

> ⚠ **It is vital that every threatening incident is reported, however minor. Otherwise a colleague may encounter a more severe incident in the same setting which could have been avoided.**

MAINTAINING PERSPECTIVE

While it is important to be aware of risk and take appropriate action to avoid it, it is equally important to maintain an objective outlook. Generally, unpleasant or threatening incidents are the exception rather than the rule for all community nurses.

It is unhelpful for an individual or family to be labelled as 'difficult' or 'aggressive', as people dealing with them in future may anticipate and even precipitate such behaviour by their expectations.

 It would be better to tell colleagues that 'on this occasion, the individual behaved aggressively' than to say 'this is an aggressive individual'.

Similarly, an area or estate may have an undeserved or exaggerated reputation for danger, and it is better to try to make an objective judgement:

• Look for the positive as well as the negative aspects of an area.
• Consider the impact of any negative aspects from the residents' point of view, as well as the visiting professionals': it is the residents who have to live with the problems.
• Ask clients about their experiences of living in the area.
• Consider whether you can help local people to overcome some of the negative aspects of life in the area: e.g. by helping them to campaign, putting them in touch with influential agencies or individuals, or bringing in ideas for successful action from other areas.
• Don't perpetuate an undeserved or exaggerated reputation about an area.

OTHER HAZARDS

Other health and safety hazards which might be encountered in the course of work in the community, such as hazardous premises or aggressive animals, should be noted and reported to colleagues. If there is a danger of actual injury, the GP, as the person responsible for the patient's care, or a community nurse manager or team leader, might need to contact the patient to discuss the impact of the hazard on the provision of care. In less extreme circumstances, other colleagues will at least be forewarned, and able to prepare appropriately.

MANUAL HANDLING

Manual handling of patients may be necessary in the course of the work of district nurses or community paediatric nurses who work with seriously ill people, or of nurses in residential units or nursing homes. There is possibly a greater risk of injury to the nurse in primary care than in a hospital setting because of restricted space, non-standard beds and mattresses and the absence of colleagues to assist. However, all districts hold a store of equipment to assist in moving and handling, such as hoists, which can be loaned to an individual for use in the home.

As in hospital settings, each Trust will have a policy on manual handling of patients, and carry out regular training and updating.

 It is essential that the manual handling policy of the Trust is followed, in all circumstances.

Nurses working for private employers, such as in nursing or residential homes, will find the provision of lifting aids such as hoists, and training, varies. If they are concerned about the circumstances under which manual handling is carried out, or their training needs are not met, they should discuss it with their employer or manager.

 Advice on health and safety can be obtained from your professional association, who can also advise on negotiating with your employer.

APPEARANCE

UNIFORM

The type or even existence of a uniform for nurses working in the community varies greatly in different parts of the country. Some areas have dropped the requirement for their community nurses to wear any uniform at all, arguing that the benefits of uniform are outweighed by the disadvantages (see Box 9.2). In other areas, some community nurses – usually district nurses – still wear a traditional uniform, while elsewhere this has been modified to allow the wearing of trousers and tunics.

Box 9.2 Advantages and disadvantages of wearing uniform

Advantages:
    Looks professional
    Saves wear and tear on own clothes
    Identifies nurse to patient/client
    Easy to launder.

$\rightarrow$

Box 9.2 *(contd)*

Disadvantages:
  Can be unsuitable for lifting etc.
  Can alienate some clients
  Makes nurse conspicuous.

Health visitors do not wear uniform, and some other groups of professionals also wear their own clothes for some or all their work: clinical nurse specialists, community mental health nurses and some practice nurses are examples.

GENERAL APPEARANCE

If a uniform is not worn, Trusts employing community nurses usually have some guidelines about appropriate appearance whilst at work. General principles are:

• Clothing should be appropriate for the delivery of care (e.g. avoid narrow skirts which might restrict lifting).
• It should not give offence to clients.
• It should be safe (see Box 9.2).
• Clothing, and jewellery and make-up, if worn, should be appropriate for a professional.

This last requirement can be the subject of differences of opinion between nurses and their employers.

 Check with the Trust policy for more detailed requirements.

SUMMARY

Some of the practical issues which need to be considered by nurses working in the community are mobility, use of the car, and health and safety, including personal safety. While it is important to recognize and avoid risk, it is equally important to maintain a clear perspective. Where community nurses are employed by Trusts, they will be able to consult Trust policies for guidance in each of these areas. Other primary care nurses will need to discuss the issues with their employers, and negotiate agreements for working practice.

Further reading

Health and Safety Commission 1987 Violence to staff in the health services. HMSO, London

10

Infection control

As with many areas of nursing practice, the principles of infection control in primary care are the same as those followed in acute hospital settings. However, primary care nurses work in a wide range of settings, which have different implications for putting the principles of infection control into practice.

INFECTION CONTROL IN DIFFERENT SETTINGS

The setting for care may be:

• People's homes – there are no facilities such as trolleys from which to undertake dressings or prepare injections. Homes vary in cleanliness, temperature and humidity, and often contain a variety of animals, birds and other humans who may pose a risk of contamination to clean materials and infection to the patient.

> **!** You should aim to give the best possible standard of care, according to the principles of infection control, in the circumstances.

• Clinics and surgeries–many people pass through these places every day, and couches, instruments and equipment are used by many people in the course of a single surgery.

> **!** You must know and put into practice the clinic or surgery procedure for cleaning, disinfecting or sterilizing instruments and equipment.

• Informal settings – some nursing care may be given in hostels, in village halls or even on the street. In these circumstances the nurse has to decide on each occasion how to follow the principles of infection control to give the best possible care.

INFECTION CONTROL AND DIFFERENT CLIENTS

As many more people with serious or terminal illness are nursed in their own homes and managed in primary care, it would be wrong to assume that infection control is less important, or that the conditions encountered by nurses in primary care are less hazardous, to nurse or patient.

Patients may be nursed at home with central venous catheters, or with impaired immunity, or with infections such as human immunodeficiency virus (HIV) or hepatitis B or C. Some doctors' surgeries are equipped to perform endoscopies and minor surgery, and contain a wide range of instruments and equipment.

The principles and areas of concern in infection control in primary care are the same as those in hospitals;

- the use of universal precautions
- cleaning and sterilizing instruments and equipment
- disposal of clinical waste
- disposal of sharps.

UNIVERSAL PRECAUTIONS

These are barrier methods which prevent contamination by blood or body fluids. They are recommended by the Department of Health for all health care workers as a matter of good practice.

> ⚠ **Adopting universal precautions means that it is not necessary to know whether or not any individual poses a biohazard threat.**

Universal precautions consist of:

- covering cuts or abrasions on exposed skin with a waterproof dressing
- wearing disposable latex or vinyl gloves when dealing with blood or body fluids

> ⚠ **Some pharmaceutical companies supply doctor's surgeries with disposable plastic gloves; these are not as strong as latex or vinyl and are prone to splitting. They should not be worn for protection against infection.**

- washing hands properly between procedures (see Box 10.1)
- wearing disposable aprons if there is a possibility of splashing by blood or body fluids

Box 10.1 Handwashing technique

- Use liquid not bar soap and warm or hot water.
- Use a sterile soft bristle brush (if available) for nails.
- Do not scrub hands as this debrides the skin.
- Remove rings as these can harbour microorganisms.
- Ensure that all surfaces of the hand are washed, including palm, dorsum and areas between the fingers.
- Dry hands thoroughly on disposable paper towels.

Adapted from the RCN guide to infection control in hospitals (RCN 1994).

- wearing eye protection if there is a danger of flying contaminated debris or blood splashes
- disposing of sharps safely (see below)
- avoiding needlestick injuries (see below)
- irrigating with copious amounts of water any conjunctiva or mucous membranes which are accidentally contaminated
- dealing appropriately with spillages (see below)
- dealing appropriately with waste (see below).

CLEANING, DISINFECTING AND AUTOCLAVING

These different techniques reduce the risk of infection to different degrees (see Box 10.2). They will be appropriate in different circumstances depending on:

- the nature of the object (e.g. what it is made of, how big it is, how it is used)

Box 10.2 Definitions regarding cleaning of instruments/equipment

- *cleaning*–removes some microbes, bacteria, viruses and fungi
- *disinfection*–reduces vegetative microbes but not bacterial spores
- *sterilization*–achieves complete destruction of microorganisms and their spores and all living matter
- *decontamination*–methods of cleaning, disinfection and sterilization for the removal of microbial contamination from equipment.

From the RCN guide to infection control in hospitals (RCN 1994).

• the degree of microbiological safety required (i.e. whether it must be sterile).

There are hundreds of different pieces of equipment in use in primary care today, and it is not possible to list them and describe the way in which they should be cleaned and/or disinfected or sterilized. In general, however:

• Single-use ('disposable') instruments should be used where they are available.
• Single-use instruments should never be cleaned/sterilized and reused.
• The manufacturer's instructions regarding cleaning and/or disposal of instruments must be followed, both for safety and legal indemnity reasons.
• Nurses working for Trusts must read and follow the Trust policy on infection control.
• Nurses employed by GPs, nursing homes or other private employers must ensure that they know who is responsible for the maintenance of instruments, and for instrument cleaning and sterilizing.

> ⚠ **Trust policies will set out procedures for dealing with contaminated instruments or equipment which has to be transported from a patient's home or other setting to a central point for decontamination.**

Nurses working in a GP's surgery who are not employed by a Trust may find that there is no written infection control policy for them to follow. In these circumstances it is even more important that the principles of infection control are followed, and the manufacturer's instructions are followed regarding the frequency and method of sterilization or cleaning of equipment. If the nurse is using instruments or equipment, she must be confident that they are safe for the patient, which will include being confident that they have been correctly cleaned or sterilized, using an appropriate and effective method.

> ⚠ **The UKCC Code of Professional Conduct states that the nurse must 'ensure that no action or omission ... within your sphere of responsibility, is detrimental to the interests, condition or safety of patients'.**

In addition to personal professional accountability, the nurse may also be responsible for supervising the infection control activities of the practice. This should include:

- getting the GP partners and staff to agree a written infection control policy
- ensuring that the practice autoclaves are serviced and tested at the recommended intervals
- ordering sufficient stocks of single-use instruments, cleaning and disinfecting materials, gloves, aprons and other protective clothing
- arranging initial training and regular updating of practice staff about infection control issues and techniques
- undertaking regular audits of practice infection control standards.

SPILLAGES OF BLOOD OR BODY FLUIDS

These should be dealt with immediately. Disposable gloves and an apron should be worn. The spillage should be completely covered with either:

- NaDCC (sodium dichloroisocyanurate) granules, or
- disposable paper towels which are then treated with 10,000 parts per million sodium hypochlorite solution (i.e. a 1:10 bleach solution). After a few minutes the spillage can be wiped up with disposable paper towels, using a gloved hand, and the towels and gloves disposed of as clinical waste.

DISPOSAL OF CLINICAL WASTE

This is an area of practice which is closely controlled by legislation. The control of Substances Hazardous to Health Regulations 1988 (COSHH) require an assessment to be carried out of the risk from clinical waste, and the Environmental Protection Act 1990 includes a duty of care regarding waste management, and a standard classification of waste, together with recommendations for its disposal (see Box 10.3).

Box 10.3 Different classes of waste and their disposal

- *normal household waste*–black plastic bags
- *clinical waste arising from direct patient care* – yellow plastic bags
- *aerosols and glassware* – brown cardboard boxes
- *soiled and infected linen* – red plastic bags
- *non-infected linen* – clear plastic bags
- *cytotoxic waste* – orange plastic containers

All Trusts and Health Authorities have policies and systems relating to the disposal of clinical waste, and nurses in primary care should ensure that they are familiar with these.

The general principles are;

• Waste which does not constitute a risk can be placed in opaque packaging, sealed and disposed of as household waste.

This 'non-risk' waste is the only waste which can be disposed of in the patient's home.

• Clinical (including potentially infected) waste should be placed in a yellow bag, sealed and placed in a suitable container until it can be transported to a disposal point.

Again, nurses employed to work in GP's surgeries may find that systems for disposal of clinical waste are not clearly defined by a written policy. If in doubt, advice can be obtained from the local Health Authority or from a Trust Infection Control Nurse Specialist with a responsibility for primary care.

DISPOSAL OF SHARPS

'Sharps' are not only needles, but also items such as glass slides, ampoules and stitch cutters. Sharps must always be disposed of in a used sharps container at the place where they have been used: it should never be necessary to carry sharps from room to room, or further. For this reason, community nurses carry special small used sharps bins with them.

It is the responsibility of the user to dispose of the sharp object in the appropriate container, and the responsibility of the employer to dispose of the container.

Some common examples of poor practice must be avoided if sharps are to be disposed of safely:

• Needles must never be resheathed before disposal.
• Needles should not be bent or cut before disposal.

• Needles should not be disconnected from syringes before disposal.

Sharps containers should comply with the British Standard Institute's regulations (BS 7320), and should not be filled more than two thirds full. When they are ready for disposal, the containers must be sealed.

NEEDLES IN THE COMMUNITY

Some patients will use needles regularly in their own homes: for example, diabetic patients who inject insulin. They can be issued with used sharps containers which comply with the British Standard, and arrangements made for the disposal of the full containers. Individuals will need to be taught initially, and reminded at intervals, of the importance of safe disposal of sharps. If specially manufactured sharps containers cannot be supplied to individuals for any reason, they are sometimes advised to use a screw-top jar instead.

> ⚠ Advice about the use of alternatives to standard used sharps boxes should always be sought from an appropriate source such as an Infection Control Nurse.

Used needles are sometimes found in the street when they have been used by drug abusers, and cause understandable concern to local communities. The local Drugs Action Team (DAT) usually has a policy for the collection and disposal of such needles, and community nurses should refer urgently to the DAT rather than collect any such needles themselves.

IMMUNIZATION FOR COMMUNITY STAFF

Immunization against hepatitis B is recommended for all health care workers, including students, who have direct contact with patients' blood or blood-stained body fluids. In addition, staff of residential accommodation for people with severe learning difficulties are considered to be at higher risk because of the higher prevalence of hepatitis B carriers among this population, as well as the perceived higher risk of bites and scratches from clients with challenging behaviour.

Nurses working for Trusts should find that this is included in the infection control policy, and dealt with by the Occupational Health Service. Nurses working for other employers, such as GPs, should discuss immunization with

their employer, and may need to obtain immunization from
their own GP.

SUMMARY

Infection control is an important topic, governed by
legislation and controlled locally by the policies of NHS
Trusts and health authorities. Nurses working for trusts
should have access to Trust policies: nurses working for GPs
and other private employers have a responsibility to ensure
that they are aware of their own local arrangements for the
safe use and disposal of instruments and clinical waste.
Infection control in a range of different settings poses different
challenges to a hospital environment, but the principles to be
applied remain unchanged.

Further reading

RCN 1994 Guidelines for Infection Control in Hospitals. Royal
College of Nursing, London
Department of Health 1996 Immunisation against Infectious
Disease. HMSO, London

Dealing with drugs in primary care

There are many situations in which nurses working in primary care are involved in the administration of medicines (see Box 11.1). The fact that their clients are not in an acute hospital setting does not mean that the drugs they are prescribed are less potent or more straightforward than those used in hospitals. In fact the relative isolation of nurses working in surgeries and people's homes means that the professional responsibility for the administration of medicines, and the associated duties to ensure safe and appropriate prescribing, administration and monitoring, are exercised with great care.

The prescription, administration, handling and disposal of drugs in the community is largely governed by the same legislation and professional guidance as drugs used in any other setting. However, there are some elements of the guidance which apply specifically to primary care, and some practical issues which arise in community settings. The degree of autonomy and control enjoyed by patients in primary care is also an important factor which must be taken into account by nurses dealing with patients' medication in the community setting.

Box 11.1 Examples of nurses' involvement with medicines in primary care

Practice nurses:
- administration of vaccines
- administration of / advice about contraceptive drugs and appliances
- monitoring of drugs with toxic side effects
- adjustments to dosages / delivery devices for insulin in diabetes and preventive and reliever drugs in asthma
- administration of nebulized bronchodilators in acute asthmatic attacks.

District nurses:
- administration of drugs in palliative care via syringe driver, injection or infusion
- administration of vaccines
- topical treatments of venous and arterial leg ulcers
- administration of insulin to housebound diabetics etc.

School nurses:
- administration of vaccines.

Community mental health nurses:
- regular administration and monitoring of depot neuroleptic drugs.

Nurse practitioners for the homeless:
- initiation of wound treatment
- monitoring of TB treatment etc.

LEGISLATION

Three pieces of legislation govern the prescription and supply of medicines:

- the Medicines Act 1968
- the Misuse of Drugs Act 1971
- the Medicinal Products: Prescription by Nurses etc. Act 1992.

The Medicines Act divides all drugs (except controlled drugs) into three categories:

- Prescription Only Medicines (POMs)
- Pharmacy Only medicines (P)
- General Sales Lists (GSL) medicines.

The Misuse of Drugs Act 1971, and later Misuse of Drugs Regulations 1985, concern particular drugs which are liable to abuse. These are classified into five 'schedules':

- Schedule 1 includes drugs such as cannabis and lysergide which are not used medicinally, and are generally prohibited.
- Schedule 2 includes drugs such as diamorphine (heroin), morphine, pethidine, amphetamine and cocaine, which can be used subject to the controlled drug requirements (see below).
- Schedule 3 includes barbiturates and other drugs which are subject to special prescription requirements but not to safe custody requirements nor the requirement to keep a register.
- Schedule 4 drugs include benzodiazepines such as diazepam which are subject neither to special prescription nor to safe custody requirements.
- Schedule 5 drugs are preparations which are subject to the minimal requirement to keep invoices relating to them for 2 years.

The most important schedules, in terms of their impact on the practice of health care professionals, are Schedule 2 (opiates and amphetamines) and Schedule 3 (barbiturates). These are 'controlled drugs', and must be handled accordingly.

NURSE HANDLING OF CONTROLLED DRUGS

! **Special provision is made for midwives to obtain and administer some controlled drugs for pain relief during labour. These are set out in detail in the UKCC's Midwives Rules and 'Midwife's Code of Practice'.**

For nurses, there are three principal areas of practice which are affected by controlled drug status:

- safe custody
- reconciliation and record keeping
- disposal.

Safe custody requirements are defined by the Misuse of Drugs Act (Safe Storage) Regulations, and apply to nursing or residential homes, and other community institutional settings such as community homes and private hospitals. Specific standards are set out for cabinets and rooms in which controlled drugs are stored. For most community nurses, working in people's homes and GP's surgeries, storage of stocks of controlled drugs will not be an issue, as the supply of controlled drugs will usually be to a named patient by prescription. The safe storage of the controlled drug by the patient is not governed by law. However, if the nurse does have possession of a controlled drug during practice, it must be kept in a locked receptacle, and be accessible only to the individual nurse. Trusts employing community nurses will have their own protocols governing these circumstances.

Reconciliation is the process of accounting for each dose of a controlled drug, and ensuring that entries in registers concerning the stock level and the usage of controlled drugs are accurate at all times. It must take place in settings where stocks of controlled drugs are held, such as hospices or community hospitals, to the following guidelines:

- Reconciliation must take place on every occasion that a controlled drug is administered, stock is received or responsibility for it changes hands.
- A controlled drug register or record book must be kept solely for this purpose.
- A separate page or section should be used for each different preparation.
- Alterations should not be made; instead mistakes should be noted and a second, correct entry made in the book.
- Records must be kept for 2 years.
- Any medicines wasted or destroyed should be accounted for during reconciliation.
- Reconciliation should be undertaken in accordance with local Trust protocols.

> ⚠ There is no legal requirement to keep a record of administration of controlled drugs *dispensed for an individual patient* other than in the patient's nursing notes or chart.

Disposal of controlled drugs which are recorded in a register (i.e. not those dispensed to an individual patient) must be witnessed by an 'authorized person': that is

- a police officer
- a Home Office inspector
- an inspector of the Royal Pharmaceutical Society
- a NHS unit Chief Executive
- a health authority medical adviser
- a regional pharmaceutical officer.

The date and quantity destroyed must be entered into the register book, and signed by both people present.

> ⚠️ **A pharmacist or medical practitioner can destroy prescribed drugs returned by a patient without making a record and without the presence of an authorized person.**

Clearly there are different procedures for controlled drugs dispensed to individual patients by prescription, and those taken from a stock of controlled drugs held by a community institution or a midwife. Nurses must ensure that they know the origin of controlled drugs, and are clear about their responsibilities in law and to their employers.

> ⚠️ **Nurses working for a Trust must ensure that they have access to an up-to-date Trust protocol relating to the administration of medicines in community settings, and that they act in accordance with it.**

OTHER CATEGORIES OF DRUGS

As well as controlled drugs, there are three other categories of drugs defined in The Medicines Act by how they can be obtained:

- Prescription Only Medicines (POMs) can only be obtained with a prescription. POMs are drugs which meet the criteria shown in Box 11.2, though other factors can be taken into account when deciding if a drug should have POM status (Box 11.3).
- Pharmacy (P) drugs can only be sold or supplied from a registered pharmacy under the supervision of a pharmacist.

Box 11.2 Prescription Only Medicine criteria

POMs are drugs which:

- could present danger, directly or indirectly, even if used correctly without medical supervision
- are frequently used incorrectly and so could present a danger to human health directly or indirectly
- contain substances, the activity or side effects of which require further investigation
- are normally prescribed parentally.

From EU Classification of Medicines Directive 1992

Box 11.3 Other factors in deciding the legal status of a drug

- the presence of narcotic or psychotropic substances in non-exempt quantities
- the risk of medicinal abuse, possibility of addiction or illegal misuse
- novel substances with properties requiring fuller investigation
- where the usage is confined to hospitals or for conditions diagnosed in hospitals
- where the use is intended for outpatients but requires specialist/special supervision.

- Drugs on the General Sales List (GSL) can be sold from other retail outlets, such as shops, although the quantities in which they can be sold can be limited.

Medicines which are sold by a pharmacist, or other retailer, without a prescription, are often informally referred to as 'over-the-counter' (OTC) medicines.

 In hospitals, it is accepted practice that all medicines are supplied only on prescription.

NURSES' ROLE WITH OVER-THE-COUNTER MEDICINES

While POMs and P medicines generally have a doctor's or pharmacist's advice dispensed with them, people may ask the advice of nurses about medicines which they have bought, or are thinking of buying, over the counter. The OTC Directory, published annually by the Proprietary Association of Great Britain, lists 18 different therapeutic categories of OTC preparations, with a number of subcategories in each. It is essential that nurses acknowledge any limits in their knowledge of these preparations, and advise patients to take advice from a pharmacist if they cannot answer questions themselves. Some general points apply to all OTCs, however:

• Encourage people to follow the manufacturer's instructions about correct dosage and usage of the remedy.
• Encourage the patient to allow OTCs sufficient time to work, in accordance with manufacturer's instructions, before assuming they are ineffective.
• Record the patient's use of OTCs so that interactions or duplications with prescribed medicines can be avoided
• Remind the patient of the availability of advice on OTC preparations from pharmacists.

NURSES' ROLE WITH ADMINISTRATION OF MEDICINES

Nurses can be involved with:

• administering a medicine
• assisting in the administration of a medicine
• overseeing self-administration by a patient.

The UKCC guidance 'Standards for the Administration of Medicines' 1992 states that under any of these circumstances nurses should be satisfied that they:

• have an understanding of substances used for therapeutic circumstances
• are able to justify any actions taken
• are prepared to be accountable for the action taken.

Specifically, this means that the practitioner must:

• be certain of the identity of the patient to whom the medicine is to be administered
• be aware of the patient's current assessment and planned programme of care
• pay due regard to the environment in which care is being given
• scrutinize carefully the prescription, where available, and the information provided on the relevant containers
• question the medical practitioner or pharmacist if information is illegible, unclear, ambiguous or incomplete, and if necessary refuse to administer the substance

- refuse to prepare substances for injection in advance of their immediate use, and refuse to administer a medicine not placed in a container or drawn up into a syringe by him or her, or in his or her presence except in specific circumstances (e.g. already established intravenous infusion, syringe pumps or other continuous infusion)
- draw the patient's attention to information leaflets concerning their prescribed medicine.

Details of the nurse's responsibilities in relation to the actual administration of the medicine are shown in Box 11.4.

Box 11.4 UKCC requirements when administering drugs

- Check the expiry date.
- Consider dosage, method, route and timing of administration in the context of the condition of the patient.
- Consider whether there may be dangerous interactions between prescribed drugs.
- Determine whether medicine should be withheld pending consultation with doctor, pharmacist or other colleague.
- Contact prescriber if contraindications to drug exist.
- Make clear, accurate, written and signed records at time of administration.
- Record if patient refuses drug.
- Use opportunity to teach patient and carers about effects and side effects of drug.
- Record positive and negative effects of drug, and make known to prescribing practitioner.
- Ensure any replaced entries on records are correctly depleted to avoid accidental duplication of medicines.

MEDICINES AND AUTONOMY IN PRIMARY CARE

An important part of the nurse's role is to explain to people the purpose, mode of action and effects of the drugs they are prescribed. People in their own homes and in charge of their own or their relatives' medication have the choice of compliance or non-compliance with the prescribed regime every time the dose is due. Understanding how the medication will help their condition, and what effects are to be expected, makes it much more likely that they will take the drug as the prescriber intended, and so gain maximum benefit.

Box 11.5 Elements of a protocol for administering drugs without an individual patient prescription

The protocol should state:

- **who** can be given the drug (i.e. which group of patients)
- **when** (in what circumstances) it can be given (i.e. assessment of patient to be carried out prior to administration of emergency drugs, or expert recommendations for vaccines for people travelling abroad)
- **what** can be given (drug, dose and route of administration)
- **how and where** the drug should be obtained (e.g. from surgery stock)
- **which staff** can administer the drug (e.g. nurse with specialist asthma training for emergency doses of nebulized salbutamol)
- **how and where** the administration should be recorded.

⚠ It is important to identify people who cannot read, because of poor literacy or poor eyesight, or cannot read English, and to ensure that they understand the purpose, action and required dosage of their medicines, otherwise the required regime for effective treatment is unlikely to be followed.

AUTHORIZATION FOR NURSES TO ADMINISTER MEDICINES

Prescription Only Medicines can only be prescribed by medical or dental practitioners. However, the UKCC Standards identify three ways in which nurses working in community practice can be authorized to administer these substances:

- by an individual patient prescription
- by a protocol setting out the arrangements by which substances can be administered to certain categories of persons who meet the stated criteria (e.g. protocols for immunization programmes). This is a facility provided by Section 58 of the Medicines Act allowing substances to be administered to a number of people in response to an advance 'direction' from a medical practitioner

> **!** The administration of medicines under protocol was subject to a Department of Health enquiry in 1996/97 and a report is expected to clarify the legality of this practice.

- by verbal authorization in a telephone conversation with a medical practitioner *only* for a single administration where it has not been possible to anticipate the need for treatment.

Examples of instances when community nurses might need an alternative form of authorization to the individual patient prescription are:

- immunization programmes (see Chapter 14)
- emergency situations (such as for the administration of nebulized salbutamol during an asthma attack).

In these instances, a written protocol must be in place covering the key issues (see Box 11.5) before any drug is administered without an individual patient prescription.

SAFETY IN HANDLING DRUGS

Some medicinal substances are irritant and/or very potent, and should be handled with particular care. These include:

- corticosteroids
- antibiotics
- phenothiazines
- cytotoxics.

Contact with the skin and inhalation of dust should be avoided. It is essential that nurses handle any drugs under their care in accordance with the manufacturer's instructions. This applies particularly to vaccines, which must be stored at the correct temperature (usually 2–8°C) in order to preserve their potency.

> **!** Vaccines which are transported by nurses (e.g. to a patient's home) must be transported in a cool-box or insulated container to ensure that the required temperature is maintained.

It is essential that nurses in primary care who travel around their community are conscious of the security of any medicines they carry. Some people assume that all doctors and nurses in the community carry supplies of drugs, and may break into cars, or steal bags from health centres, hoping to find drugs which can be used or sold on. For this reason, some Trusts advise their nurses not to display 'Nurse Visiting' signs in their cars. It is important not to leave bags or boxes in sight in a car when it is unattended.

> ⚠ The UKCC guidance on Administration of Medicines states that 'where a practitioner working in the community becomes involved in obtaining prescribed medicines for patients, she or he must recognize her or his responsibility for safe transit and correct delivery'.

SAFETY WITH DRUGS IN THE HOME

Nurses in primary care deal with people who are usually living at home. They are therefore in an ideal position to advise on safe handling of medicines, and so minimize accidents, drug wastage and accidental drug misuse.

Clients should be advised to:

- keep all medicines out of the reach of children
- keep medicines in the original, usually child-resistant containers
- take particular care with medicines dispensed in strip or blister packaging
- always finish the prescribed course of medicine, unless subsequently advised against this by their doctor (e.g. because of side-effects, a change in medication or a change in diagnosis)
- refrain from sharing prescribed medicines with other people
- return any unwanted medicines to their local pharmacist for destruction.

DRUGS AND CHILDREN

Children differ from adults in their response to drugs, particularly in the neonatal period. Dosages are calculated according to body weight or body surface area in very young children, and by body weight or age in older children.

> **!** It is a legal requirement for a doctor to write the age of a child under 12 years on a prescription, and good practice to state the age on all prescriptions for children.

When an oral liquid preparation is prescribed for a child, and the dose is smaller than 5 ml, an oral syringe is supplied with the medicine. The syringe is marked in 0.5 ml divisions from 1 to 5 ml, and is provided with an adaptor and instruction leaflet. Parents or carers of young children should be advised to use the syringe for both extracting the dose from the container, and delivering the medicine orally to the child.

> **!** Parents should be advised NOT to add medicines to a child's feeding bottle or plate, since the drug may interact with the milk or food, and the dose may be reduced if the milk or food is not finished.

DRUGS AND OLDER PEOPLE

Older people often have particular issues related to medicines, such as:

- polypharmacy
- physical difficulties
- inappropriate prescribing
- increased susceptibility.

Polypharmacy refers to the common situation in which an older person is prescribed or acquires a range of different medicines for different ailments. This can lead to confusion and accidental misuse of the medicines, as well as increased risk of side effects and drug interactions.

There are a number of actions a community nurse can take to help:

- Ensure that the person has a written record of all their drugs which can be shown to the different health professionals they visit or are visited by.
- Ensure that the individual (or carer if they take responsibility for helping with medicines) understands what each of the drugs is for, and how it should be taken.
- Encourage the person to have their medicines regularly reviewed by their GP or pharmacist, by, for example, taking their written medicines list to consultations.

• Remind them to include in their list any over-the-counter medicines they take, since these can also cause interactions or side effects.
• Ask the prescribing GP to add descriptive wording to the prescription which will be reproduced on the label by the pharmacist, to help distinguish different tablets (e.g. 'The Sedative Tablets').

Physical difficulties for older people can include: difficulty in gaining access to their medicines, particularly if they are dispensed in child-resistant containers; difficulty with labelling and instructions because of poor eyesight; and difficulty in swallowing tablets or capsules. Nurses can help by advising the patient or carer:

• to ask for medicines to be dispensed in non-child-resistant containers
• to obtain special aids designed to help remove screw tops from jars (advice from an occupational therapist might be helpful)
• to ask for large-print labels on medicine bottles
• to take tablets or capsules with plenty of fluid
• to ask for medicines to be prescribed in liquid form if available.

Inappropriate prescribing can occur when the natural consequences of ageing, such as loss of postural stability, or of social circumstances, such as bereavement, lead to the prescribing of further medicines. Sometimes social support, advice or adaptations to home or lifestyle are more appropriate responses than medicines. Increased susceptibility to the effects of drugs occurs in older people because of reduced renal clearance, which causes drugs to be excreted more slowly. Acute illness can further reduce renal clearance, so the metabolism of drugs will be affected by infections and other illnesses. Tissue concentrations of drugs may be increased by as much as 50%. Adverse reactions are then more common, and may have significant consequences for more vulnerable older people:

• Mental confusion, caused by many commonly used drugs, may lead to concerns among family and carers about the onset of age-related dementia.
• Constipation, caused by antimuscarinics and many tranquillizers, can cause considerable distress and lead to self-medication or further prescribing.
• Postural hypotension, caused by diuretics and many psychotropic drugs, can lead to falls which may cause fractures and other injuries.

Nurses in primary care need to be alert to the effects of medication, and consider these when assessing an older person's nursing or social needs. They also need to act as advocate for the individual with other health professionals, ensuring that all medication, including self-medication, is entered into client records, and is regularly reviewed for suitability and effectiveness.

MONITORING DRUGS

As well as administering drugs, nurses in primary care can be involved in monitoring the progress of people on particular medications. Common conditions requiring blood monitoring of their therapeutic regimes are:

- epilepsy
- thyroid dysfunction
- rheumatoid arthritis
- respiratory conditions treated with theophylline
- blood clotting disorders treated with warfarin.

Practice nurses or district nurses may be involved in collecting blood specimens and completing appropriate request forms. The interval between tests will be determined by a monitoring protocol, previous results and the condition of the patient.

> **!** **Nurses involved in monitoring of drug levels should have access to a protocol setting out the monitoring regime, the tests required and action to be taken on receipt of results.**

NURSE PRESCRIBING

The prescribing of some medicinal products by nurses was suggested in the Cumberlege Report 'Neighbourhood Nursing – A Focus for Care' in 1986. It was not until 1992 that the Medicinal Products: Prescription by Nurses etc. Act became law, and the pilot programme of nurse prescribing began in 1994. There were eight demonstration sites in England, in which nurses who held a health visiting or district nursing qualification undertook additional training before beginning to prescribe from a limited list of drugs and products. Nurse prescribing is due to be extended to all nurses with a health visiting or district nursing qualification, who undertake additional training. The list of items which nurses can prescribe remains limited, however, and in the near future the major part of the nurse's role in medication will be in administration and advice to patients.

THE ROLE OF THE PHARMACIST IN THE COMMUNITY

There are two types of pharmacist who work in the community: the community services pharmacist (CSP), and retail pharmacists.

Each district has a community services pharmacist, whose remit is to advise staff working in primary care on drug issues. The CSP is often involved in ordering and supplying vaccines for childhood immunization programmes, and can advise on new vaccines and the appropriate storage and transport of vaccines, as well as providing rapid warning of any public health concerns over vaccine safety and efficacy. They may also be involved in training courses for community nurses undertaking immunization.

> **!** The CSP can usually be contacted through the pharmacy department of the local hospital Trust.

Retail pharmacists are business people who run 'chemist' shops, though they usually prefer to be referred to as pharmacists and pharmacies. Part of their income is derived from the dispensing fee they receive for handling NHS prescriptions. The opening of new pharmacies is controlled by health authorities, and restrictions apply to prevent a proliferation of pharmacies in some areas, and the neglect of other areas. The health authority's role is to protect the patients' interest by ensuring that everyone has reasonable access to a dispensing service.

In recent years pharmacists have expanded their professional role to include more than the packaging and dispensing prescription of medicines. Some pharmacists now also undertake:

- medicine reviews for people taking multiple medications
- collection of prescriptions from GPs' surgeries and delivery of medicines to patients' homes
- advice about minor conditions such as colds, skin complaints, or head lice
- screening tests for high blood lipids or blood sugar
- other tests such as blood pressure measurement
- advice about healthy eating, exercise and smoking cessation.

> **!** The rising costs of prescriptions, and the increasing workload and therefore waiting time in GPs' surgeries, means that people are more willing to ask the advice of a pharmacist about minor ailments and their treatment.

135

Box 11.6 Pharmacists' Code of Ethics

Principles:

1. A pharmacist's prime concern must be for the welfare of both the patient and other members of the public.
2. A pharmacist must uphold the honour and dignity of the profession and not engage in any activity which may bring the profession into disrepute.
3. A pharmacist must at all times have regard to the laws and regulations applicable to pharmaceutical practice and maintain a high standard of professional conduct. A pharmacist must avoid any act or omission which would impair confidence in the pharmaceutical profession. When a pharmaceutical service is provided, a pharmacist must ensure that it is efficient.
4. A pharmacist must respect the confidentiality of information acquired in the course of professional practice relating to a patient and the patient's family. Such information must not be disclosed to anyone without the consent of the patient or appropriate guardian unless the interest of the patient or the public requires such disclosure.
5. A pharmacist must keep abreast of the progress of pharmaceutical knowledge in order to maintain a high standard of professional competence relative to his sphere of activity.
6. A pharmacist must neither agree to practise under any conditions which compromise professional independence or judgement nor impose such conditions on other pharmacists.
7. A pharmacist or pharmacy owner should, in the public interest, provide information about available professional services. Publicity must not claim or imply any superiority over the professional services provided by other pharmacists or pharmacies, must be dignified and must not bring the profession into disrepute.
8. A pharmacist offering services directly to the public must do so in premises which reflect the professional character of pharmacy.
9. A pharmacist must at all times endeavour to cooperate with professional colleagues and members of other health professions so that patients and public may benefit.

In these areas pharmacists are clearly working alongside the primary health care team, and usually have some regular contact with local GPs and staff. Some health professionals are concerned about the calibration and quality of equipment used for screening in pharmacies, and about the level and appropriateness of the training given to counter assistants who may be involved in giving advice. It is important that any concerns are raised at practice or primary health care team meetings, so that the pharmacy in question can be contacted, and constructive dialogue can be initiated.

THE PHARMACISTS' CODE OF ETHICS

The Royal Pharmaceutical Society has agreed a Code of Ethics for pharmacists which combines nine 'principles' with more detailed 'obligations'. These guide the pharmacist in the delivery of a professional service, and could be used to judge the validity of any concerns from members of the primary health care team. The principles are set out in Box 11.6.

SUMMARY

Nurses in primary care are involved in the prescribing, administration and monitoring of medicines. They are also expected to be able to advise people about self-medication. Some groups of people, such as older people and children, require additional care and advice. Nurses also work with community and retail pharmacists, who are increasingly involved with medication issues.

Further reading

BMA/RPS 1997 British national formulary. BMA/The Pharmaceutical Press, London – reprinted frequently

OTC directory. Proprietary Association of Great Britain – reprinted annually

DoH 1996 Immunisation against infectious disease. Department of Health, London

UKCC 1992 Standards for the administration of medicines. UKCC, London

UKCC 1993 Midwives rules. UKCC, London

UKCC 1991 A midwife's code of practice. UKCC, London

RPS 1997 Medicines, ethics and practice – a guide for pharmacists. Royal Pharmaceutical Society, London

SECTION 3

Preventive activity

12

Health promotion work

The term health promotion is used to mean many different things (see Box 12.1). A general and practical definition might be 'activities, including information giving, which aim to help people look after their health'. Nurses in primary care have always been involved in health promotion work, as well as providing health care when needed, because of the long-term and holistic nature of their contact with individuals and families. This chapter provides an overview of this work.

STRATEGIES FOR HEALTH

'HEALTH OF THE NATION'

The first Government 'strategy for health' of recent years was 'The Health of the Nation', published in 1992. It identified five key areas for action to protect and improve people's health:

- coronary heart disease and stroke
- cancers
- accidents
- HIV/Aids and sexual health
- mental health.

Targets were set in each area for measurable improvements (see Box 12.2). Each district health authority aimed to reduce the prevalence figures in its population to the required levels,

---

Box 12.1 Definitions of health promotion

- 'The process of enabling people to increase control over, and to improve, their health' (World Health Organization, Alma Ata Declaration, 1978).
- 'the main components of health promotion: prevention, health education and healthy public policy' (Linda Jones 'The rise of health promotion' in Katz & Peberdy (1997)).
- 'an umbrella term for a very wide range of activities which enhance good health and well-being and prevent ill-health. It includes: health education and health information; preventive medical measures (such as screening clinics and immunization); healthy public policies (such as regulations about smoking in public places); environmental measures which improve health and safety (such as traffic calming and the provision of good, affordable housing); community and organizational health development (enabling communities and organizations to identify and meet their needs for better health)' (Simnett 1995).

Box 12.2 'The Health of the Nation' targets

CHD and stroke:
- to reduce death rates for both CHD and stroke in people under 60 by at least 40% by the year 2000
- to reduce the death rate for CHD in people aged 65–74 by at least 30% by the year 2000
- to reduce the death rate for stroke in people aged 65–74 by at least 40% by the year 2000.

Cancers:
- to reduce the death rate for breast cancer in the population invited for screening by at least 25% by the year 2000
- to reduce the incidence of invasive cervical cancer by at least 20% by the year 2000
- to reduce the death rate for lung cancer under the age of 75 by at least 30% by the year 2000
- to halt the year-on-year increase in the incidence of skin cancer by the year 2000.

Mental illness:
- to improve significantly the health and social functioning of mentally ill people
- to reduce the overall suicide rate by at least 15% by the year 2000
- to reduce the suicide rate of severely mentally ill people by at least 33% by the year 2000.

HIV/AIDS and sexual health:
- to reduce the incidence of gonorrhoea by at least 20% by 1995
- to reduce by at least 50% the rate of conceptions amongst the under-16s by the year 2000

Accidents:
- to reduce the death rate for accidents among children aged under 15 by at least 33% by 2005
- to reduce the death rate for accidents among young people aged 15–24 by at least 25% by 2005
- to reduce the death rate for accidents among people aged 65 and over by at least 33% by 2005.

using a combination of methods. These included broad, public health approaches as well as action by individual health professionals with individual patients.

'OUR HEALTHIER NATION'

A consultation document on a new strategy for health was published in 1998. 'Our Healthier Nation' built on 'The

Health of the Nation', but reduced the number of specific targets to just four (see Box 12.3).

Three settings were identified for action to reduce the impact of heart disease and stroke, cancers, mental health and accident; they were:

- healthy schools (focusing on children)
- healthy workplaces (focusing on adults)
- healthy neighbourhoods (focusing on older people).

Box 12.3   'Our Healthier Nation' Green Paper targets

- Heart disease and stroke – to reduce the death rate from these conditions in people aged under 65 years by a third
- Accidents – to reduce the incidence of accidents, defined as a visit to a GP or A+E as a result of injury, by at least a fifth
- Cancer – to reduce mortality from cancer in people aged under 65 years by at least a fifth
- Mental health – to reduce mortality from suicide and undetermined injury by at least a sixth.

HEALTH PROMOTION IN ACTION

Five different approaches to health promotion, including population and professional action, are shown in Box 12.4.

Box 12.4   Approaches to health promotion

- Medical – the promotion of medical interventions to prevent or ameliorate ill-health
- Behaviour change – changing people's attitudes and so their behaviour in order that they adopt healthier lifestyles
- Educational – giving information about cause and effects of ill health and helping people develop skills for healthy living
- Client-centred – working with issues, choices and actions identified by clients, and empowering the client
- Societal change – taking political or social action to change the physical or social environment

Adapted from Jones and Naidoo, 1997

PREVENTION OF ILLNESS

Preventing ill health is a basic component of all of these approaches. Prevention activities are often broken down into those which constitute 'primary prevention', 'secondary prevention' and tertiary prevention':

• 'Primary prevention' aims to prevent the onset of disease. One example of this is immunization.
• 'Secondary prevention' aims to detect and treat disease at an early stage, so as to prevent it causing more major harm. Screening for cervical cancer is an example of this, as the early, pre-cancerous lesions detected through screening can be treated, and the malignant disease prevented.
• 'Tertiary prevention' aims to minimize the effect of a disease, or slow its progression. The education, monitoring and care of people with diabetes is an example of tertiary care.

HEALTH PROMOTION AND NURSES IN PRIMARY CARE

Most nurses in primary care have an element of 'one-to-one' or group health promotion in their work. For example:

• District nurses help patients to change their diet to avoid constipation when taking morphine-based painkilling drugs.
• Health visitors discuss the benefits of breastfeeding with mothers.
• Practice nurses teach diabetic patients how to monitor their own blood glucose levels.
• School nurses discuss ways to protect sexual health with adolescents.

ONE-TO-ONE AND GROUP HEALTH PROMOTION

The resources necessary for these are essentially the same. They are:

• space and time
• equipment
• information resources
• training/preparation.

Steps to setting up a health promotion session:

• Identify a room, or arrange to spend time with a patient at home, preferably when they will not be distracted or interrupted, for example, by the need to care for small children at the same time.

• Gather appropriate resources: for a session on smoking cessation you might want an ecolyser, which demonstrates the level of carbon monoxide in the blood, smoking diaries, dummy nicotine replacement patches to show the patient, or other resources.

• Collect information to give to patients: if you are helping a mother plan a healthy diet for her vegetarian teenagers, you will need appropriate leaflets, videos, telephone helpline numbers, local support group contact, and/or other sources of help and support.

• Ensure that you know enough about the topic, by attending study sessions, gaining appropriate qualifications, undertaking distance learning or private study.

Running group sessions requires some additional skills. These include:

• helping a group to form and define its membership
• ensuring that the group 'task' – learning, sharing, practising, etc. – is completed
• making sure all members of the group are heard, and their views respected, and that no member dominates or disrupts the group
• keeping the 'boundaries' of the group, so that members do not stray into tasks or discussions which are not part of the reason for the group.

These are not skills which most people naturally possess, and group skills training can be very useful.

WHOLE-POPULATION HEALTH PROMOTION

Health visitors in particular also take a more public health approach to health promotion, by working for changes at community level which will improve or protect the health of whole populations, not just individuals. An example would be a campaign to have a dangerous road crossing moved, or a heavily polluted piece of land cleaned up. Such work requires experience, political sensitivity and the ability to work effectively with a range of different statutory and voluntary organizations. It is an area in which new or inexperienced community nurses would need to work alongside more experienced colleagues.

HEALTH PROMOTION IN GENERAL PRACTICE

The 1990 GP Contract encouraged a more structured approach to health promotion in general practice. This part of the Contract has been modified twice since 1990 (see Box 12.5), and most general practices now undertake a programme of health promotion which:

> **Box 12.5** Health promotion in the GP contract
>
> • 1990 – health promotion on any topic, patients to be seen in clinics of ten or more, payment to the practice per clinic. Criticized for encouraging quantity rather than quality, and for not attempting to target health promotion at major causes of illness or death.
>
> • 1993 – 'banding' system replaced clinics: practices could choose which band to enter. Band one focused on data collection about smoking habits, and activity to assist smoking cessation. Band two included band one activities, with the addition of data collection and activity on detecting hypertension in the practice population. Band three included smoking and hypertension, with the addition of information about obesity, exercise and family history in the data collection, and health-promoting activities on these topics. Focused on CHD and hypertension, major causes of illness and death, but criticized for setting targets on data collection which detracted from time available for health promotion activities.
>
> • 1995 – banding discontinued and replaced by health promotion programmes designed by each practice individually. Programmes had to focus either on a Health of the Nation priority, or on a priority for the practice population, and had to be approved by a local Health Promotion Committee.

• focuses on the particular needs of the practice population
• sets measurable objectives
• is reported on annually to the health authority.

Much of the health promotion work carried out with individual patients, or groups of patients, in general practice is undertaken by nurses: often the practice nurse, and sometimes the district nurse, health visitor or school nurse.

HEALTH PROMOTION IN OTHER SETTINGS

Programmes have been set up in a variety of settings which aim to protect and improve the health of the people in those settings. The commonest examples are:

• health-promoting schools – in which schools 'sign up' to a number of health-promoting measures, such as banning smoking on school premises, displaying health education literature, and formulating policies on health issues such as asthma;

• health-promoting workplaces – in which employers agree to health-promoting measures such as allowing health screening during working hours, restricting smoking, providing measures to combat work-related injuries, and identifying sources of health information and support for staff.

HEALTH PROMOTION PROTOCOLS

Health promotion activity undertaken by nurses is often carried out using a protocol – guidance to the professional undertaking the consultation or session on what should be included, what information or resources are given to the patient, when investigation, treatment or referral is indicated, and other important parameters. The advantages of using a protocol are:

• All professionals involved give the same service to patients, on each occasion. *Example*: the GPs, nurses and health visitors all immunize babies using the same injection site, so the parents do not worry that one of them was 'wrong' if different sites are used.
• All patients have equal access to information, investigation and referral. *Example*: patients with abnormal blood pressure are asked to return for further monitoring at the same interval regardless of whether they see the nurse or the GP, so they do not assume their condition has worsened if they are brought back earlier by a different professional.
• The service is based on 'best practice' guidelines rather than individual practice. *Example*: diabetes mellitus is diagnosed at the nationally recognized level of fasting blood glucose, rather than at different levels used historically by the practice.
• A nurse 'filling in' on a clinic or consultation for an absent colleague knows exactly what is usually done. *Example*: patients attending for a contraceptive clinic have the same checks and examination undertaken before prescriptions are issued, so they do not lack confidence in the locum nurse.

The Royal College of Nursing has issued guidelines for the development of protocols (see Box 12.6). The most important aspect of protocol development is the involvement of all parties who will be using the protocol in its development. Protocols which are imposed by one professional group on another are unlikely to be useful, or even used. Sample protocols, which can be adapted to the needs of a particular practice or group of nurses, can be obtained from various sources, including other surgeries, Medical Audit Advisory Groups or Primary Care Audit Groups (contacted through health authorities) and professional organizations. Wherever it originates, a good protocol will be:

• specific to the practice or nurses using it
• agreed by all concerned

> **Box 12.6** Royal College of Nursing guidelines on protocol development
>
> * The purpose of the protocol is explicit.
> * The protocol is founded on research.
> * The protocol is not a replacement for individualized care planning.
> * A protocol is devised only when there is a need to assist nurses and other health professionals to deal with complex operational issues.
> * All those who are required to follow the protocol should be involved in its production, either directly or through their representatives.
> * All parties or their representatives should agree to the contents of the protocol.
> * Any party to the protocol has the right to seek a review at any time.
> * The protocol should be reviewed regularly and whenever there is a change of circumstances.

* practical and achievable
* reviewed regularly.

SUMMARY

Promoting health and preventing ill health are areas of work which feature in recent national health policy documents. Most nurses in primary care are involved in some aspect of health promotion, whether through work with individuals, groups of patients or whole communities. Where more than one nurse is involved, or when a complex range of investigations and referrals are undertaken, protocols enable nurses to take a structured approach to health promotion activity which ensures equity, quality and safety for the client.

Further reading

Department of Health 1992 The health of the nation: a strategy of health for England. HMSO, London

Department of Health 1998 Our healthier nation – a consultation document. The Stationery Office, London

Scriven A, Orme J (eds) 1996 Health promotion – professional perspectives. The Open University, Milton Keynes

Jones L, Naidoo 1997 Theories and models in health promotion. In: Katz J, Peberdy A (eds) Promoting health – knowledge and practice. The Open University, Milton Keynes

Simnett I 1995 Managing health promotion – developing healthy organisations and communities. Wiley, Chichester

13

Cervical screening

Cervical screening is screening designed to detect pre-cancerous changes in the cervix uteri which might, if untreated, lead to malignancy. It is an example of secondary prevention – that is, prevention which aims to detect and treat disease at an early stage – rather than primary prevention, which is intended to prevent a disease occurring. Practice nurses carry out most of the cervical screening undertaken in general practice, while nurses working in community cytology clinics and family planning clinics also perform cervical smears. Other nurses in primary care, such as health visitors, are involved in giving information to women about cervical screening, to encourage their attendance.

> ⚠ **Cervical screening is the process of taking a sample of cells from the cervix to examine for pre-cancerous changes before any symptoms are experienced.**

CERVICAL CANCER

Cancer of the cervix uteri (neck of the womb) causes the death of around 1700 women in England every year. In 1991, 19,000 women in England and Wales were found on screening to have pre-cancerous cells in the cervix. These are the cells which can develop, over a period of 10–15 years, into malignant cells, although they may also regress spontaneously. If treated at this pre-cancerous stage, these cells can be completely removed. Nurses involved in cervical screening need to understand:

- the anatomy of the cervix
- the technique for obtaining a satisfactory sample of cells from the cervix for examination – the 'smear'
- the meaning of different findings on the cytological report
- the functioning of the National Cervical Screening Programme.

THE ANATOMY OF THE CERVIX

The cervix forms the lower third of the uterus (this is why it is called the 'cervix uteri'). It is cylindrical in shape and 2.5 cm in length. The 'internal os' of the cervix opens into the body of the uterus, and the 'external os' opens into the vagina (see Figure 13.1). The cervix is made up of fibrous connective tissue and smooth muscle, lined with epithelium. In the

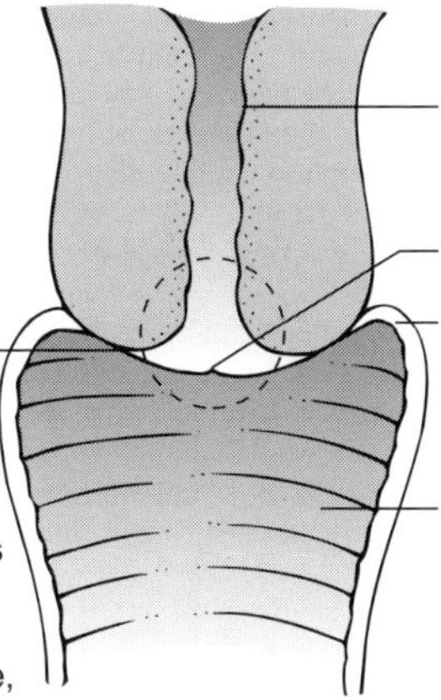

Fig 13.1 Anatomy of the cervix.

endocervix (usually just inside the cervix) the lining is columnar epithelium, which changes to squamous epithelium in the ectocervix (the part next to the vagina). As this 'transformation zone' is the place from which cervical cancer is thought to arise, it is from this area of the cervix that cells need to be obtained for a satisfactory smear. The actual anatomical position of this area varies: in post-menopausal women, it may be inside the external os, while in women with 'ectropian' – an eversion, or turning out, of part of the cervix – it may be visible when the cervix is visualized.

> ⚠ **The most important aspect of successful cervical screening is ensuring that the correct cells are collected in the sample.**

TAKING A CERVICAL SMEAR

The Royal College of Nursing has issued guidelines for nurses involved in taking cervical smears. The RCN emphasize the importance of all nurses having appropriate training before undertaking this procedure, and recommend that they have access to the British Society for Clinical Cytology video and publication 'Taking Cervical Smears' (see 'Further reading'). Equipment needed for taking a cervical smear includes:

- a couch or bed with a blanket or sheet for cover, in a room which is private and protected from interruptions
- a good light source which can be adjusted as necessary
- vaginal speculae, usually Cusco's, either metal (requiring sterilisation following use) or disposable plastic
- wooden spatulae, usually Ayres' or Aylesbury, and/or cytobrush for collecting sample of cells from the cervix (see figure 13.2).
- a glass slide, labelled with the woman's details, fixative solution, and a slide box for tranporting the sample to the cytology laboratory, together with appropriate laboratory request form
- disposable latex gloves (these do not need to be sterile). Assessment of the patient before undertaking the smear should include:
- details of recent menstrual history (first day of last period, any irregular bleeding)
- contraceptive use (as this may influence the appearance of the cervix or the cells on the smear)
- any history of abnormal smears or treatment for cervical abnormality
- any fears or concerns about the procedure, so that these can be addressed before proceeding.

The procedure for taking a smear involves the following steps:

- The woman should be encouraged to empty her bladder

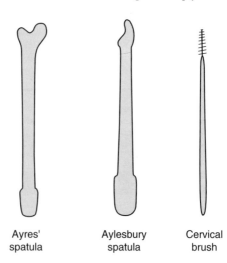

Ayres' spatula   Aylesbury spatula   Cervical brush

Fig 13.2 Examples of spatulae used to take samples for cervical cytology.

before the examination starts, then remove her clothing below the waist.

• She usually lies on her back, with knees drawn up and legs spread, feet together. She should be covered with a sheet until the smear is about to be taken. If the woman is obese, it is sometimes easier to take the smear with the woman in the left lateral position, and using a Sims speculum.

• The light is positioned low down so that it can illuminate the cervix once the speculum is in place.

• The speculum can be warmed with water if necessary, but is not lubricated with jelly as this can affect the appearance of the cervical cells on examination. It is inserted gently in the closed position, then opened to allow the cervix to be seen. It is essential that the cervix is visible before the smear is taken, both to allow any abnormalities to be observed, and to ensure that the smear is taken from the appropriate area.

• With the speculum in place and the cervix visible, the longer point of the spatula is gently inserted into the external cervical os, and rotated through 360 degrees, to ensure that cells from the squamo-columnar junction – the 'transformation zone' – are sampled.

• The spatula is withdrawn and the sample is immediately spread onto the glass slide with a stroking motion, and covered with the fixative solution. Exposure to the air begins to alter the cells, so immediate fixing is essential. If the cytobrush is used to obtain a sample, the instructions supplied by the manufacturer for its use should be followed.

• After the procedure, the woman is allowed privacy to dress before being informed of the procedure for obtaining the results of the test, and having any further questions answered.

> ⚠ Taking a cervical smear is an invasive and intrusive procedure for which the woman's consent should always be explicitly obtained.

INTERPRETING THE CYTOLOGY REPORT

The pre-cancerous changes on the cervix are known as cervical intraepithelial neoplasia (CIN). The appearance of the cells scraped from an area of CIN is called dyskaryosis, and is usually classified by the cytology laboratory as borderline or mild, moderate or severe. Actual cancerous cells are described as invasive carcinoma, or glandular neoplasia, and need further investigation, usually by colposcopy, to confirm a diagnosis of cervical cancer. Different results as described on the laboratory form, and the recommended actions, are shown in Table 13.1.

Table 13.1
Examples of cervical cytology results and suggested actions[a]

Result code	Explanation	Action
Inadequate	Insufficient cells on slide/ Inadequately fixed/ Obscured by blood/	Repeat smear
Negative	Normal–may include simple inflammation	Routine recall
Borderline changes	Nuclear changes which may be dyskaryotic	Repeat at 6 months
Mild dyskaryosis	Cellular appearances of CIN 1	Repeat at 6 months
Moderate dyskaryosis	Cellular appearance of CIN 2	Refer for colposcopy
Severe dyskaryosis	Cellular appearance of CIN 3 (?carcinoma in situ)	Refer for colposcopy
Severe dyskaryosis ?invasive Ca	Appearance of CIN 3 and ?invasive carcinoma	Refer for colposcopy
Glandular neoplasia	Suggests cancer or pre-cancer in cervical endometrium	Refer for colposcopy

[a]Based on Austoker & McPherson (1992)

The following figures give some idea of the likelihood of an abnormal result:

• In 1994/95, 91% of smear tests were reported as 'negative'.
• Of the abnormal smears, around 7% showed borderline or mild dyskaryosis (CIN 1), 1.7% showed moderate or severe dyskaryosis (CIN 11), and only 0.2% suspected invasive cancer or glandular neoplasia (CIN 111).

> **!** **All women should be informed of their results in writing, whether negative or positive.**

GIVING RESULTS

If a woman's result is not straightforward – for example, if the smear needs to be repeated because the sample was inadequate – a personalised letter, with an explanatory leaflet or note, is more appropriate than a form letter. An early appointment with, or an opportunity to telephone and speak to the doctor or nurse should be offered. A woman may assume that any result which is not clearly negative is in fact positive for cancer, and great distress can be caused by insensitive handling of results. When the result does show an abnormality which needs further investigation, such as colposcopy, or treatment, the nurse should follow the clinic or surgery protocol in deciding who should discuss this with the woman.

> **!** **Colposcopy is a microscopic examination of the cervix using a colposcope, during which the cervix can be stained so that abnormal cells show up.**

It is useful to have a set of leaflets or information sheets in the surgery or clinic about the meaning of different results. A woman may not remember much of a verbal explanation, particularly if she is tense or distressed, and written information to take away can be more effective.

THE NATIONAL CERVICAL SCREENING PROGRAMME

Cervical screening began in Britain in the mid-1960s, but the national NHS Cervical Screening Programme was set up in 1988. All health authorities were instructed to introduce computerized call and recall systems, based on lists of women registered with local GPs, in order to invite those aged 20–64 for screening at least once every 5 years. Individual districts can decide to screen more frequently, based on local health needs assessment, and some screen every 3 years.

> **!** **Women who have had a hysterectomy involving removal of the cervix are excluded from the national cervical screening programme.**

The screening programme is a collaborative undertaking, depending for its success on high standards of practice from all organizations and individuals involved in the process:

- health authorities, who need to keep up-to-date lists of women registered with each GP in their district, adding women as they reach the age of 20 and removing women who reach 65, handing on women who move out of the district to their new health authority, and receiving those who move in
- GPs and nurses in primary care, who need to encourage women to attend, maintain their own competence through training and audit of their practice, take adequate smears from the correct area of the cervix, and ensure that women are informed of the results and referred on for investigation and treatment as necessary
- cytology screeners, who review the slides in the laboratory, and need to accurately identify and report abnormalities.

> ⚠ **A national coordination office based in Sheffield is responsible for maintaining and improving the quality of the National Cervical Screening Programme.**

CERVICAL SCREENING IN GENERAL PRACTICE

Since the 1990 GP contract, GPs have received payments if the percentage of women registered with them who have had a cervical smear in the previous 5 years reaches a particular level. There is a lower payment if 50% of eligible women have been screened, and a higher payment if 80% have been screened. These payments act as an incentive to practices to encourage women to attend for screening. Since 1990, many more smears have been taken in general practice, and in some areas community-run cytology clinics have performed far fewer smears as a result. Closure of these clinics reduces women's choice about where to go for screening, particularly if they do not want to attend their family doctor's surgery.

There are a number of groups of women who are disadvantaged by the national screening programme as it is currently run:

- women not registered with a GP, which can include for example homeless women, or people with learning disabilities living in group homes, who will not be included on lists held by the health authority and so not invited for screening

- women who do not have a normal postal service, for example, on some travellers' sites, as call and recall, and notification of results, is carried out by letter
- homeless women and those in temporary accommodation or short-term refuges, as having no address, or frequent changes of address, means call-up and results letters cannot be delivered
- women who are not able to read, as they have to rely on others to read information, appointment letters and results
- women who do not read or speak English, as they have to rely on others to read and interpret appointment letters, information and results.

SUMMARY

Cervical cancer can be prevented by treating cells in the precancerous stage. The National Cervical Screening Programme relies on the cooperation of health authorities, GPs and nurses in primary care and laboratory cytology screeners to undertake successful screening of women aged 20–64. However, some women are disadvantaged by this system, and their needs must be considered by nurses who come into contact with them.

Further reading

Austoker J, McPherson A, 1992 Cervical screening, 2nd edn. Oxford Medical Publications, Oxford

BSCC 1989 Taking cervical smears. British Society for Clinical Cytology, London

NHSCSP 1966 Cervical screening: a pocket guide. NHS Cervical Screening Programme, London

RCN 1994 Cervical screening: guidelines for good practice. Royal College of Nursing, London

14

Immunization

Immunization has been responsible for dramatic decreases in the morbidity and mortality associated with a range of infectious diseases. National immunization programmes, particularly those aimed at children, rely heavily on the involvement of community nurses, both in carrying out the immunization, and in educating people about immunization:

- Practice nurses give many of the childhood immunisations, as well as having a key role in vaccinating travellers abroad and managing and delivering influenza vaccination programmes.
- Health visitors are responsible for initiating the childhood immunization programme by discussing immunization with mothers, and, if appropriate, obtaining initial consent for the child to be included in the immunization programme. Health visitors who work with elderly people will also be involved in the influenza programme.
- District nurses are involved in ensuring that people on their caseload with chronic illnesses are vaccinated against influenza.
- Nurses working with vulnerable groups, such as people with learning disabilities or mental illness, and homeless people, ensure that their clients receive appropriate vaccinations, for example, against hepatitis B.
- School nurses work on the childhood immunization programme, both educating children about the need for immunization, and participating in immunization sessions.

> ⚠ **Immunization is an example of primary prevention, which aims to prevent disease from occurring, rather than to treat or minimize the effects of existing disease.**

TYPES OF IMMUNITY

'Immunization' is the process of conferring immunity to a disease. 'Vaccination' refers to the process of giving a vaccine in order to confer immunity.

Immunity can be active or passive, and natural or 'acquired' – also called 'artificial' immunity (see Table 14.1). The vaccination programmes in which community nurses are involved give a person artificial immunity, which may be:

- active – when a vaccine is given to stimulate an immune response (i.e. antibody production) from the body: this type of immunity is usually long-term

Table 14.1
Different types of immunity

	Natural	Artifical
Active	Antibodies produced by stimulation of immune response during infection	Antibodies produced by stimulation of immune response by vaccine
Passive	Antibodies passed from an immune person to a recipient, e.g. via placenta	Antibodies from an immune person given to recipient, e.g. by injection of gammaglobulin

- passive – when antibodies from a person who is already immune are injected into another person, and the recipient does not produce antibodies: this type of immunity is usually short-term, lasting only a matter of weeks.

VACCINES

The vaccines which are used to confer immunity consist of components of the infecting organism which have been altered to prevent them causing the disease itself. They may be:

- inactivated, i.e. killed (e.g. rabies vaccine)
- attenuated, i.e. live but weakened (e.g. polio vaccine, measles, mumps and rubella vaccine, and BCG vaccine)
- split, i.e. containing parts of the infecting organism (e.g. influenza and pneumococcal vaccine)
- toxoids, i.e. containing toxins produced by the organism which have been inactivated (e.g. tetanus and diphtheria vaccines).

Vaccines will only be effective if they have been stored correctly – in a vaccine refrigerator, and protected from light – and they are used in accordance with manufacturer's instructions. The storage and transport of vaccines at the correct temperature (usually 2–8°C) is referred to as 'maintaining the cold chain'. An immunization coordinator in each health district has overall responsibility for immunization programmes, and the maintenance of the cold chain will be overseen by this individual.

For nurses in primary care, the storage and transport of the vaccine is within their sphere of responsibility while it is within the clinic or surgery, or being transported to patient's homes. They should ensure that vaccines are handled in the manner recommended by the manufacturers, and the guidance in the Department of Health handbook 'Immunisation against Infectious Disease' (see Box 14.1).

Box 14.1 Guidelines for storage of vaccines

• Vaccines should be stored in a refrigerator specially designed for the storage of medicinal products (domestic fridges are not suitable).
• Food and drink should not be stored in the same refrigerator, to avoid frequent opening of the door.
• The temperature of the vaccine fridge should be monitored and recorded regularly, preferably daily, using a maximum and minimum thermometer, which will indicate if the temperature has been above or below that recommended at any time.
• Vaccines should never be allowed to freeze, as they may deteriorate and the container may crack.
• Cool boxes or insulated containers should be used to transport vaccines.
• Multi-dose vials of vaccine should not be kept beyond the end of an immunization session.
• Electricity supplies to vaccines fridges should be protected by physical means and/or warning notices to avoid accidental interruption of the supply.

CHILDHOOD IMMUNIZATION

The current childhood immunization programme aims to immunize children against the following diseases:

• tetanus
• diphtheria
• pertussis (whooping cough)
• poliomyelitis
• *Haemophilus influenzae* type B infections
• measles
• mumps
• rubella
• tuberculosis.

The current schedule of primary courses (which stimulate immunity) and boosters (which maintain immunity) is shown in Table 14.2.

Table 14.2
The childhood immunization schedule (1998)

Vaccine	Age
Diphtheria/tetanus/pertussis (DTP) Polio (oral) and Hib	1st dose 2 months 2nd dose 3 months 3rd dose 4 months
Measles/mumps/rubella (MMR)	12–15 months
Booster DT and Polio (oral) MMR 2nd dose	3–5 years
BCG	Infancy or 10–14 years
Booster tetanus/diphtheria Polio (oral)	13–18 years

> **!** **Department of Health guidance says: 'It is every child's right to be protected against infectious diseases. No child should be denied immunisation without serious thought as to the consequences.'**

Children with asthma, chronic lung and congenital heart conditions, Down's syndrome or HIV infection, and premature or small for dates babies, are at increased risk of complications from infectious dieseases, and these children should be immunized as a matter of priority. Children with no spleen, or no functioning spleen, are also at increased risk from bacterial infections. In addition to the scheduled vaccines, they should also have pneumococcal vaccine, influenza vaccine, meningococcal A and C vaccine. Children on renal dialysis need hepatitis B vaccine.

> **!** **Premature babies should be immunized from 2 months after birth, regardless of the extent of prematurity.**

IMMUNIZATION BY NURSES

Department of Health (1996) guidance states that:

> *'A doctor can delegate immunisation to nurses if three conditions are fulfilled:*

- *the nurse is willing to be professionally accountable for this work as defined in the UKCC guidance on the 'Scope of Professional Practice'*
- *the nurse has received training and is competent in all aspects of immunisation, including the contraindications to specific vaccines*
- *adequate training has been given in the recognition and treatment of anaphylaxis (see Chapter 28).*

If these conditions are fulfilled, and nurses carry out the immunisation in accordance with accepted District Health Authority, NHS Trust or Health Board policy, the Authority/Trust/Board will accept responsibility for immunisation by nurses. Similarly, nurses employed by GPs should work to agreed protocols including all the above conditions'.

Practice nurses and their employing GP should ensure that they have written surgery protocols in place for childhood immunizations, in order to fulfil these criteria. Health visitors should have a copy of their Trust protocol relating to immunizing children.

> ⚠ **Joint training for all nurses involved in immunization programmes is helpful to ensure that practice is consistent no matter which professional carries out an immunization, and that parents receive consistent advice.**

IMMUNIZING CHILDREN

It is important to check manufacturer's instructions before administering a vaccine. Generally, the following guidance applies:

- All vaccines in the childhood programme, except BCG and oral polio vaccines, are given by injection.
- BCG is always given by intradermal injection; all other injectable vaccines are given by deep subcutaneous (SC) or intramuscular (IM) injection.
- A 23 or 25G needle should be used for immunizing infants.
- In infants, injections should be given into the anterolateral aspect of the thigh, or the upper arm; if the buttock is used, the upper outer quadrant should be used to avoid damage to the sciatic nerve.
- If the skin is cleaned (some protocols do not include skin cleaning) then alcohol must be allowed to evaporate before injection of vaccine as it can inactivate live vaccine preparations.

• Hold the child's limb firmly to ensure the injection is given in the correct site – encourage the accompanying adult or a colleague to hold the child on their lap for comfort and safety.

CONSENT TO IMMUNIZATION

> **⚠ Consent must always be obtained before immunization. Written consent provides a permanent record, but written or verbal consent is required at the time of each immunization, after the child's fitness and suitability have been established.**

A child under 16 may give consent for immunization, provided he or she understands fully the benefits and risks involved. Where a child under 16 who fully understands the benefits and risks wishes to refuse the immunization, that wish should be respected.

WHEN SHOULD VACCINES *NOT* BE GIVEN?

Contraindications to vaccines vary, and the manufacturer's instructions for each vaccine should be checked. However, there are some general contraindications, both systemic and local to the injection site, which are shown in Box 14.2. Children with complex histories, and particularly those currently undergoing treatment for serious illnesses, may have special needs. Their consultant or GP will prescribe appropriate vaccines at appropriate times.

Box 14.2 General contraindications to immunization

- acute illness on day of immunisation
- history of severe local or general reaction to preceding dose:
  - severe local reaction: extensive area of redness and swelling which becomes indurated and involves most of the anterolateral surface of the thigh or a major part of the circumference of the upper arm;
  - severe general reaction: fever equal to or more than 39.5°C within 48 hours of vaccine; anaphylaxis; bronchospasm; laryngeal oedema; generalized collapse. Prolonged unresponsiveness; prolonged inconsolable or high-pitched screaming for more than 4 hours; convulsions or encephalopathy occurring within 72 hours.

OTHER CONCERNS

The media often report controversy about the immunization of children, with varying reports of vaccine injury, association of vaccine with the development of chronic illnesses, or concern about the origin of vaccines. Nurses involved in vaccination need to be aware of these reports, and prepared to discuss the risks and benefits of immunization with parents and older children. Department of Health guidance in 'Immunisation against Infectious Disease' includes references for some of the controversial studies, as well as guidance from expert groups about immunizations. When parents have questions or concerns beyond the scope of the nurse's knowledge, they can be referred on to their child's GP, the district Immunization Coordinator or a consultant paediatrician for further advice.

> **!** **The Council for the Faculty of Homeopathy strongly supports the immunization programme, and has stated that immunization should be carried out in the normal way using the conventional tested and approved vaccines, in the absence of medical contraindications.**

ADULT IMMUNIZATIONS – GENERAL

There is no national programme of immunizations for all adults, as there is for children. Most immunizations for adults are given for one of two reasons:

- to maintain immunity acquired through the childhood programme, by giving 'booster' doses, or
- to protect against the risk of other diseases, not covered by the childhood programme, which may affect the individual.

BOOSTERS

Tetanus is caused by the toxin of the tetanus bacilli which enters the body at the site of an injury, particularly one involving soil or manure. Tetanus vaccine is often given as a 'booster' in adulthood. In the past, there has been a tendency to give a booster with every injury. Current guidance from the Department of Health states that this is not necessary, and can cause considerable local reactions. Tetanus boosters should only be given in certain, clearly-defined circumstances:

- if the last dose of the primary, three-dose course, or the reinforcing dose, was more than 10 years prior to an injury; or
- if a patient was not previously immunized, or their immunization status is not known, when they should have a full, three-dose course.

> **⚠** For immunized adults who have received five doses of tetanus vaccine (as in the childhood immunization programme), booster doses are not recommended, other than at the time of a tetanus-prone injury (see Box 14.3).

Box 14.3 Definitions of a 'tetanus-prone injury' (DoH 1996)

- any wound or burn sustained more than 6 hours before surgical treatment of the wound or burn
- any wound or burn at any interval after injury that shows one or more of the following characteristics:
  - a significant degree of devitalized tissue
  - puncture-type wound
  - contact with soil or manure likely to harbour tetanus organisms
  - clinical evidence of sepsis.

Tetanus booster, if given, consists of one dose of 0.5 ml adsorbed tetanus vaccine by IM or deep SC injection. Previously unimmunized adults require a course of three doses of 0.5 ml adsorbed tetanus vaccine, with intervals of 1 month between doses. Two reinforcing doses will be needed at intervals of 10 years to complete the five-dose course and ensure lifelong protection.

Patients with tetanus-prone wounds may be given human tetanus immunoglobulin, which confers rapid, short-lasting, passive immunity. 250 international units (iu) is given by IM injection, or 500 iu if more than 24 hours have elapsed since injury, if there is a risk of heavy contamination, or following burns. Human tetanus immunoglobulin is available in 1 ml ampoules containing 250 iu.

IMMUNIZATION AGAINST SPECIFIC DISEASES

Excluding vaccines given to people travelling abroad, specific vaccines are given to adults to protect against influenza, hepatitis B, meningococcal disease and pneumococcal disease.

INFLUENZA

Influenza illness is most often caused by the influenza A or influenza B viruses. Both viruses are liable to change, producing different subtypes which can cause epidemics because the population is not immune to them. Influenza vaccine is specially manufactured each year to contain inactivated strains of the viruses most likely to be circulating in the following winter. The vaccine gives 70–80% protection, and needs to be given annually.

High-risk groups, for whom vaccination is recommended, are children or adults who have:

- chronic respiratory disease, including asthma
- chronic heart disease
- chronic renal failure
- diabetes mellitus
- immunosuppression due to disease or treatment, including an absent or non-functioning spleen.

Immunization is also recommended for those living in nursing homes, residential homes, and other long-stay facilities.

> ⚠ **Immunization is not recommended for fit children and adults, including health care workers, as a routine measure.**

For adults and children aged 13 and over, the vaccine is given as a single dose of 0.5 ml by IM or deep SC injection. The vaccine should be allowed to come to room temperature and shaken well before administration.

Children aged 4–12 need two 0.5 ml doses, with the second 4–6 weeks after the first if receiving influenza vaccine for the first time. Children aged 6 months to 3 years need two 0.25 ml, with the second 4–6 weeks after the first, if receiving the vaccine for the first time. The deltoid muscle of the arm is the recommended site for adults and older children. The anterolateral aspect of the thigh is the preferred site for infants and young children.

Immunization is usually carried out in October or early November in order to protect for the following winter.

HEPATITIS B

Hepatitis B is transmitted by blood and by sexual contact, as well as by contaminated needles. The severity of the disease ranges from inapparent infection to fulminating disease with hepatic necrosis, and a 1% fatality rate. 2–10% of infected people become carriers of the hepatitis virus, and may develop progressive liver disease.

Vaccination against hepatitis B is recommended for the following groups:

- babies born to mothers who are chronic carriers of hepatitis B virus
- intravenous drug misusers
- individuals who change sexual partners frequently, particularly homosexual and bisexual men, and male and female prostitutes
- close family contacts of a case or carrier
- haemophiliacs
- people with chronic renal failure
- staff and residents of residential accommodation for people with learning disabilities
- other occupational risk groups, e.g. embalmers
- prisoners

> **!** **Immunization against hepatitis B is recommended for health care workers, including students and trainees, who have direct contact with patients' blood or blood-stained body fluids, or patients' tissues.**

The vaccine consists of a course of three 1 ml doses, with the second dose 1 month after the first, and the third 6 months after that. The preferred injection sites are the deltoid in adults, and the anterolateral aspect of the thigh in infants.

> **!** **The buttock must not be used for hepatitis B vaccination, as vaccine efficacy may be reduced.**

80–90% of people respond to the vaccine. Antibody levels can be checked by a blood test: 100 miu/ml is considered protective, and less than 10 miu/ml is considered a non-response to the vaccine. People with this level of response 2–4 months after vaccination may be offered a repeat course, and, if still unresponsive, will require immunoglobulin for protection after exposure (see below). People with antibody levels of 10–100 miu/ml can be offered a booster dose. There is no clear schedule for booster doses for people with adequate response to the vaccine, but one booster after 5 years is thought to be sufficient.

After known exposure to the virus, hepatitis B immunoglobulin (HBIG) can be given, preferably within 48 hours, to confer short-lasting, passive immunity. The dosage is 500 iu for adults and 200 iu for newborn babies.

MENINGOCOCCAL DISEASE

Meningococcal meningitis and septicaemia are caused by *Neisseria meningitidis*. Group B strains of these organisms are the commonest cause of meningitis, with Group C strains causing another third of reported infections. Group A strains are rarer in Britain. Meningitis is the commonest presentation of meningococcal disease, with 3–5% mortality. Septicaemia has a 15–20% mortality rate. The currently available meningococcal vaccine protects against Group A and Group C organisms only. Vaccination is recommended for the following groups:

- immediate family and close contacts of cases of Group A or Group C meningitis (in addition to chemoprophylaxis)
- those involved in local outbreaks in closed or semi-closed communities such as schools (advice will be available from local public health physicians)
- people travelling to sub-Saharan Africa and India for more than a month, especially if living or working with local people.

 Saudi Arabia requires immunization against meningococcal disease for people travelling to the Haj annual pilgrimage.

The vaccine is given as a single dose of 0.5 ml by deep SC or IM injection, for both adults and children. More than 90% of recipients respond to the vaccine, and immunity lasts 3–5 years.

 Routine immunization with meningococcal vaccine is not recommended, as the overall risk of meningococcal disease is very low; most infections in the UK are caused by Group B organisms, and many Group C infections occur in children too young to be protected by the vaccine.

PNEUMOCOCCAL DISEASE

Invasive pneumococcal disease includes pneumonia,

bacteraemia and meningitis. The pneumococcus is the commonest cause of pneumonia acquired in the community. One in a thousand adults is affected by pneumococcal pneumonia each year, and the mortality rate is 10–20%. Vaccination is recommended in anyone aged 2 or over who is at greater risk of pneumococcal infection due to:

- asplenia or severe dysfunction of the spleen
- chronic renal disease or nephrotic syndrome
- immunodeficiency or immunosuppression (including HIV infection)
- chronic heart, lung or liver disease
- diabetes mellitus.

The vaccine is given as a single 0.5 ml dose by SC or IM injection, preferably into the deltoid or lateral aspect of the thigh. Reimmunization is not required for most recipients, but may be necessary after 5–10 years in individuals with impaired immunity such as a malfunctioning spleen: discussion with a haematologist is advised.

 Reimmunization can cause severe reactions, especially if within 3 years of the first dose, and is not recommended.

TRAVEL VACCINATIONS

People travelling abroad may be exposed to infections which are not common in Britain. It is common practice for travel agents, holiday brochures and other sources to advise potential travellers to consult their doctor about immunization against infectious diseases before travelling. Most GP surgeries provide advice on staying healthy abroad as well as giving the specifically recommended vaccinations.

The commonest diseases included in these vaccination schedules are:

- typhoid
- hepatitis A
- yellow fever.

More rarely, immunization is needed against conditions such as rabies, tick-borne encephalitis, Japanese B encephalitis, and other diseases. Detailed information and vaccination schedules for these as well as the commoner diseases are contained in the Department of Health handbook 'Health Information for Overseas Travel'. As the recommendations change in response to local situations, a number of journals aimed at GPs and practice nurses publish regularly updated charts, usually produced by Departments of Tropical Medicine, listing travel destinations and current recommendations. Malaria chemoprophylaxis is also recommended for some travellers, and these recommendations are also included in the charts.

> ⚠️ It is essential that nurses giving advice or vaccinations to travellers refer to current authoritative recommendations for immunization schedules.

TYPHOID

Typhoid fever is a systemic infection caused by bacillus and usually spread by contaminated food or drink. Of the two hundred cases notified to the authorities in England and Wales each year, over 80% are acquired abroad. Vaccination is advised for:

- laboratory workers handling specimens which may contain the organism
- travellers to countries in Africa, Asia, Central and South America and the Caribbean, as well as some countries in Eastern Europe.

Three different typhoid vaccines are available:

- whole cell vaccine – two doses, 4–6 weeks apart, with a booster dose every 3 years; first dose must be given by deep SC or IM injection; subsequent doses can be given intradermally to reduce the severity of adverse reactions
- Vi polysaccharide vaccine: single dose by IM or deep SC injection, with booster dose every 3 years to maintain immunity
- oral Ty 21a vaccine: one capsule taken orally for 3 days, on alternate days, on an empty stomach, with a cool drink.

HEPATITIS A

Hepatitis A is most commonly spread from person to person, though contaminated food or drink may be involved. It is generally a mild disease, but fulminant hepatitis may occur. Hepatitis A is more prevalent in countries outside Northern and Western Europe, North America, Australia and New Zealand, although 80% of cases are contracted in the UK.

Vaccination is recommended for:

- travellers to areas where sanitation and food hygiene are likely to be poor

- patients with chronic liver disease
- haemophiliacs
- laboratory workers working with the virus
- homosexuals.

 Unlike hepatitis B, routine immunization against hepatitis A is not recommended for health workers.

Immunization consists of one dose of the vaccine (1440 ELISA units (1 ml) of the HM 175 strain, or 160 Antigen units (0.5 ml) of the GBM strain). It is given by IM injection in the deltoid region. This confers protection for at least one year. A booster dose at 6–12 months will give immunity for up to 10 years, and may be recommended to regular travellers.

 Hepatitis A vaccine should not be given into the gluteal region, as vaccine efficacy may be reduced.

Short-term, passive immunity can be given by the administration of human normal immunoglobulin (HNIG). This may be used as an alternative to active immunity in people who only travel occasionally. Dosage depends on body weight on the following regimen:

- for adults, travelling for 2 months or less: 0.02–0.04 ml/kg
- for adults, travelling for 3–5 months: 0.06–0.12 ml/kg

YELLOW FEVER

Yellow fever is an acute infection spread by the bite of an infected mosquito. It occurs in tropical Africa and South America. In non-indigenous, unimmunized adults the mortality rate during epidemics exceeds 50%. Immunization is recommended for:

- people travelling through infected areas
- people travelling outside urban areas in the 'endemic zone' (specific maps are contained in the regularly updated guidance)
- people requiring a certificate of vaccination for entry into a country.

> ⚠️ **Some countries require International Certification of Vaccination before allowing travellers to enter. Details can be obtained from updated guidance or the relevant embassy.**

Yellow fever vaccine consists of a single dose of 0.5 ml, given by deep SC or IM injection. It is almost 100% effective, and immunity lasts for 10 years.

> ⚠️ **Yellow fever vaccination is only given at designated Yellow Fever Centres, some of which are GP practices, and costs are borne by the recipient.**

SUMMARY

Immunization is a primary prevention activity in which most community nurses are involved. While children's immunization programmes are coordinated nationally, adults may require vaccination on an ad hoc basis depending on their health, lifestyle, and occupational risk. Nurses undertake immunization under clearly defined circumstances which include the use of a protocol and specific training in both immunization, vaccines and resuscitation.

Further reading

Department of Health, Welsh Office, Scottish Office, DHSS (Northern Ireland) 1996 Immunisation against Infectious Disease. HMSO, London
UK Health Departments and the PHLS Communicable Disease Surveillance Centre Health Information for Overseas Travel. HMSO, London [Includes lists of Yellow Fever Centres]
WHO 1998 International travel and health: vaccination requirements and health advice. World Health Organisation, Geneva [Updated annually]

15

Contraception

Many community nurses have a role in advising about contraception. Clearly, family planning clinic nurses spend most of their time dealing with sexual health and requests for contraceptive advice. But other nurses in primary care also need to give contraceptive advice:

• Many practice nurses also hold family planning clinics, as well as giving emergency contraceptive advice and treatment.
• Health visitors advise families about sexual health amongst other issues, particularly when they are involved with mothers with young children.
• Nurses working with people with learning disabilities or mental illness, or homeless people, also have to be able to advise on contraception and access to full contraceptive services.

> ⚠ **Remember that men as well as women may seek contraceptive advice, and clients may be of any age and in different degrees of mental and physical health. Contraception is not solely an issue for 'well women'.**

SETTINGS FOR CONTRACEPTIVE CONSULTATIONS

The settings in which contraceptive advice is given can vary. Community family planning clinics and doctor's surgeries provide the most common settings, but clients may also be seen in their own home, at 'drop in' centres or more informal settings. There are special family planning clinics for young people, such as Brook Advisory Centres, and other 'young person's advice clinics' at which contraception is one of a range of services offered. Whatever the setting, it is important that the necessary resources for giving people information about contraceptive choices are available (see Box 15.1).

> ⚠ **Contraceptive services are one of the few services which people can obtain from a GP with whom they are not registered.**

Not all GPs offer contraceptive services, so the service is treated as a separate item from the rest of the 'general medical services' which GPs automatically provide to all their registered patients. This means that a patient seeking contraceptive advice can 'register' with a different GP solely

> **Box 15.1** Resources for a consultation about contraception
>
> *Context*:
> - private room
> - adequate time
> - trained nurse
> - relaxed atmosphere.
>
> *Practical*:
> - examination couch
> - light source
> - sphygmomanometer etc.
> - record card/notes.
>
> *Teaching*:
> - information leaflets
> - samples of IUDs, condoms etc.
>
> Note: these resources may not be available in all circumstances, but they should be available in clinics and surgeries.

for contraceptive services. This is particularly useful for people who do not want to discuss the issue with their own doctor. Nurses involved in giving contraceptive advice in a general practice setting need to ensure that there is a valid registration form, signed by the patient, for anyone receiving contraceptive services from the practice.

 All prescriptions for contraceptive items are currently dispensed without charge to the patient.

TRAINING

The appropriate training for nurses providing full contraceptive services (advice, choices, examination and fitting of certain forms of contraception) is the ENB 901 Family Planning in Society course (or equivalent in Scotland, Wales and Northern Ireland).

Other nurses, whose role is more limited (for example, giving advice and information only) will need to ensure that their knowledge is regularly updated and that they are competent to discuss the issues raised. This may involve attendance at an 'Introduction to family planning' course, or updating sessions, or other preparation.

METHODS OF CONTRACEPTION

Contraception refers to any method designed to control fertility. In practical terms, contraception divides into two categories: planned and emergency contraception.

PLANNED CONTRACEPTION

Factors affecting choice of method

Planned contraception, by definition, is considered in advance, and so involves information and choices. Many factors can affect a person's choice of contraceptive method:

Client-related factors

• Age – an older person may choose a longer-term or even permanent method of contraception.
• Health or concerns about health – some pre-existing conditions (such as hypertension) or risk factors (such as history of thrombosis) are contraindications to some types of contraception; some people also have particular concerns, founded or unfounded, about certain methods, and so choose to avoid them; avoiding sexually transmitted disease might be as important as preventing pregnancy, so some methods will be more appropriate than others.
• Finance/career/lifestyle – condoms are the only form of contraception which is not always provided free of charge, so the cost may weigh against this method of contraception; the relative importance of avoiding pregnancy for career or lifestyle reasons will dictate how reliable a method needs to be.
• Beliefs about sex and conception – religious or cultural norms may make some forms of contraception unacceptable.
• Pattern of sexual activity – the frequency of sexual activity, and the sexual practices undertaken may influence the kind of contraceptive needed.

External factors

• Health scares and advertising – reports in the media can have a significant impact on people's choice of contraception, and advertising by companies producing male or female condoms also tries to influence choice.

• Advice from informal sources – the experience of friends and relatives can be a powerful influence on people's beliefs and choices.
• Advice from health professionals – this is highly valued by the public, so it is essential that nurses are fully conversant with contraceptive methods, their contraindications, reliability and possible side effects.
• Accessibility of services/advice/devices – people living in remote areas, or without transport, or those with physical or mental disabilities may find it difficult to reach the usual sources of advice and information, and this may limit their choice of contraception; low levels of literacy, poor understanding of language, memory problems or chaotic lifestyles may also make some forms of contraception less appropriate than others.
• Attitude of partner or family – the strength, permanency, exclusivity and nature of the relationship between the client and their sexual partner or partners will also influence their choice of contraceptive method.

> **⚠** The client needs time, information, advice and support to choose the right method of contraception.

Types of planned contraception

Contraceptive methods take different forms and can be categorized by the mechanism of their action:

• Hormonal forms alter the balance of circulating hormones to prevent conception.
• Mechanical forms prevent implantation of the fertilized ovum.
• Barrier forms prevent sperm from reaching the ovum.
• Chemical forms damage or destroy sperm.
• Surgical forms prevent passage of the ovum or sperm.
• Natural forms use the body's hormonal cycle to avoid fertile times, or avoid the deposition of sperm in the vagina.
• Combination methods use two or more methods to increase reliability.

The range of methods available in each category is shown in Table 15.1.

Efficacy

> **⚠** The efficacy of a contraceptive method is expressed as the percentage of sexually active women who would not become pregnant if they used the method according to instructions for 1 year.

Table 15.1
Methods of contraception

Category	Type
Hormonal	Combined oestrogen/progestogen pill Progestogen only pill (POP) Injectable (Depo-Provera/Noristerat) Implants (Norplant)
Mechanical	Intrauterine devices
Barrier	Diaphragm Cervical cap Male/female condom
Chemical	Spermicidal creams
Surgical	Vasectomy / female sterilization
Natural	Ovulation monitors Symptothermal method Urinary hormone monitor (Persona) Withdrawal
Combination	'Double Dutch': pill + condom Condom + spermicidal cream Intrauterine system: IUD + hormone

The efficacy of a method of contraception is sometimes described as its 'reliability' in preventing pregnancy. There are two elements which influence the reliability of any contraceptive method: the method itself (used as instructed); and the user.

'Method failure' occurs when the contraceptive fails to prevent pregnancy: for example, the intrauterine device does not prevent a fertilized ovum implanting.

'User failure' occurs when the person using the contraceptive method fails to follow the instructions for that method: for example, by omitting to take a daily contraceptive pill. Table 15.2 shows some examples of possible user failure for different forms of contraception.

Part of the nurse's role in contraception is to help people avoid user failure by:

- helping them to choose a method they understand and want to use
- giving them all relevant information, preferably in written form
- teaching the correct use of the method chosen, and allowing supervised practice if appropriate (e.g. inserting diaphragm)

Table 15.2
User failure potential in contraception

Type	User action required	Method efficacy	User failure potential	Suitable for
OCP/POP	Regular (daily) pill taking	99%	Forget to take pill	People with regular lifestyle; needing high certainty of avoiding pregnancy
Injectable	Attend for 12-weekly injection	99%	Cannot/does not attend for injections	People who cannot remember or do not want daily pill taking
Implants	Attend once for implant	99%	None	People who do not want to take regular pill or attend regular appointments
Intrauterine device / intrauterine system	Attend for fitting; check regularly for 'tail' in vagina	98–99%	Fail to notice if expelled	People who cannot take hormones; willing to check internally
Diaphragm/cap	Insert before sex; clean after use	92–96%	Fail to insert; damage by fingernails etc.	People who cannot take hormones; willing to delay/anticipate sex

Contraception
Methods of contraception

Table 15.2 (Contd)
User failure potential in contraception

Type	User action required	Method efficacy	User failure potential	Suitable for
Condoms	Insert-put on before sex	98%(male) 95%(female)	Fail to use; damage by fingernails, lubricants, etc.	People who want protection against STDs; people who do not want contact with family planning services; people who do not need very high protection
Spermicidal creams	Insert before sex	75% approx.	Fail to use	People who cannot / will not use other methods
Sterilization	Consent to op.	>99%	None	People who will never want pregnancy
Natural methods	Take temperature, check cervical mucus, test urine for hormones, etc.	94–98%	Miss daily checks, fail to abstain during fertile period	People who cannot use other methods for any reason

- ensuring that they have access to further advice and supplies whenever necessary.

EMERGENCY CONTRACEPTION

This is contraception needed after sexual activity has resulted in the possibility of unwanted pregnancy. It can be requested after omission of usual contraceptive precautions, when the normal method has failed or when sexual activity was unplanned (including sexual assault and rape).

Emergency contraception can be obtained from:

- any GP who provides contraceptive services
- a family planning clinic
- a young persons' clinic or Brook Advisory Centre
- some hospital accident and emergency departments
- some genito-urinary clinics (GUM or 'Special' clinics).

It is important to remember that women requesting post-coital contraception may be embarrassed, distressed or traumatized, and if they encounter obstacles to obtaining treatment, they may give up rather than persevere. In particular, any surgery or clinic offering this form of contraception should:

- advertise the fact on posters and surgery leaflets
- train reception staff to recognize requests for information or appointments, which may be made in obscure ways, and to deal sensitively with requests for such appointments
- ensure that at least part of the reception area can be used for private conversation with clients
- have a protocol which ensures that requests for post-coital contraception are treated as urgent, and that any woman who has had post-coital contraception is offered a follow-up appointment to discuss planned contraception.

There are two methods of 'post-coital' contraception: one hormonal and one mechanical.

The post-coital 'pill'

Emergency hormonal contraception consists of two doses of oestrogen and progesterone, given 12 hours apart. This regime can be started up to 72 hours after intercourse, and is 90–95% effective at preventing implantation.

> ⚠ It is important not to refer to this as the 'morning after' pill, as this suggests to clients that it is only effective if taken in the first 12 hours.

It is important to tell a client using this that it will not protect her from previous or future episodes of unprotected sex, and if possible a planned method of contraception should be agreed.

The intrauterine device

The second form of emergency contraception involves the insertion of an intrauterine device, up to 5 days after ovulation or the date of unprotected sex. It works by preventing implantation, and is almost 100% effective. It has the advantage of also providing a continuing form of contraception, but if the woman wishes to have it removed, this is done during her next period.

The choice between the two methods belongs to the client, but may be influenced by:

- the availability of a doctor trained to fit an intrauterine device
- access to a chemist or dispensing general practice
- plans for future fertility.

CONSULTATIONS ABOUT CONTRACEPTION

Sexual activity and contraception are very personal issues, and people may feel vulnerable and exposed when discussing them. In addition, nurses may find it difficult to discuss such issues with some clients, particularly if the age, sex, sexual orientation or sexual practices of the client fall outside the nurse's own norms. Appropriate training, giving the nurse confidence in both her/his technical knowledge and skills, and interpersonal skills for dealing with sensitive issues, are essential.

> ⚠ **The sensitivity of the subject must not lead to the consultation being rushed or curtailed, or important areas for discussion could be missed.**

During any consultation about contraceptive choices, the following issues need to be addressed:

- client's past medical history
- past contraceptive history
- female client's menstrual pattern and childbearing status
- client's views about pregnancy, now and in future
- other factors affecting choice: e.g. need for discretion, type and frequency of sexual activity, need for protection against sexually transmitted diseases

- client's current knowledge and beliefs about different contraceptive methods
- discussion of all available choices, their pros and cons, and possible side effects and reliability
- physical examination of factors such as blood pressure and weight, and discussion about lifestyle factors such as smoking and exercise
- discussion and agreement about method of choice.

It may take more than one consultation for the client to arrive at a decision about the method of choice: he or she may wish to take home information leaflets about some of the choices in order to discuss them with someone else.

Some methods can be started as soon as the client has made a decision (e.g. condoms or the diaphragm). For others it is necessary to wait for the first day of a woman's menstrual period (e.g. the contraceptive pill or injectable contraception), or another date, such as a date for surgical sterilization. In these cases it is important to discuss a temporary form of contraception, such as condoms, to protect the client in the interim.

CONFIDENTIALITY

Confidentiality is important in any clinical consultation, but may be of particular concern to some clients, such as young people, in consultations about contraception. For this reason, clients attending community family planning clinics are asked their permission before their GP is informed about their contraceptive consultation.

SUMMARY

There are many different forms of contraception, and most nurses working in primary care have some role in advising or giving information to clients on this subject. It is essential that nurses who provide contraceptive services have adequate training to do so. In this area, as many others, it is important that services are tailored to the needs of the clients who use them.

Further reading

Belfield T 1996 Contraceptive handbook–a guide for professionals. Family Planning Association, London

BMA 1994 Confidentiality and people under 16. British Medical Association, London

FPA 1997 Factsheet 12: Young people, confidentiality and the law. Family Planning Association, London

16

Chronic disease management

Chronic disease management refers to the monitoring of conditions such as asthma and diabetes in order to give appropriate advice and information to patients, to make any necessary adjustments to treatment, and to promote their best possible health. It is a tertiary prevention activity, aiming to minimize the effects of a disease, rather than to prevent disease.

Nurses in primary care are frequently involved in the care of people living with chronic conditions. For example:

• District nurses may assist people with diabetes who are housebound and cannot manage their own insulin injections and blood monitoring.
• Community children's nurses work with families whose child is living with a chronic, sometimes life-shortening condition.
• Community mental health nurses support people living with mental illness and receiving treatment and support in their own homes.
• Practice nurses run clinics in GPs' surgeries for people with chronic conditions, ensuring that they are regularly reviewed.

Many more people have chronic conditions than present to the health service with acute illness, so it is not surprising that community nurses spend more of their time dealing with these conditions. It is an area of work in which partnership with patients is the key to effective practice.

> **!** The UKCC Code of Professional Conduct states: 'As a registered nurse, midwife or health visitor, you must ... work in an open and cooperative manner with patients, clients and their families, foster their independence and recognise and respect their involvement in the planning and delivery of care'.

CHRONIC DISEASE MANAGEMENT IN GENERAL PRACTICE

As part of the 1990 GP contract, GPs were encouraged to set up health promotion clinics, including those dealing with chronic conditions such as diabetes and asthma. When the health promotion arrangements were modified in 1993, asthma and diabetes were separated from the rest of health promotion activities, and guidelines were set for the content of 'chronic disease management programmes' in general practice. These programmes continued following the changes to health promotion systems in practice which were introduced in 1995. Practices applying for payment for running chronic disease management programmes have to have arrangements in place which include:

- a register – identifying the patients in the practice who have the condition
- a call and recall system – to ensure that all known patients are regularly invited to the surgery for monitoring and health checks
- patient education – to help people understand their condition and its treatment, and their own contribution to managing it
- continuing patient education – to ensure that information given is reinforced and questions can be addressed as they arise
- protocols for clinical procedures – setting out what will happen in chronic disease consultations, which investigations will be performed at which intervals, and what action will be taken in response to monitoring
- referral arrangements – both from the nurse running the clinic to the GP, and from GP to secondary care consultants or other professionals
- appropriate personnel and training – to ensure that nurses and doctors involved in the care of patients with chronic conditions have sufficient appropriate expertise and updating
- record keeping – so that patients' progress and condition can be tracked
- audit – to measure the effectiveness of the chronic disease management programme.

> **!** These elements must be in place for a practice to claim payment from the health authority for chronic disease management of asthma and diabetes.

Although asthma and diabetes care programmes are the only ones for which a practice can claim payment from the health authority, the elements of the programme could equally be applied to the management of other chronic conditions. Conditions which would benefit from such an organized approach are shown in Box 16.1.

APPLYING THE PRINCIPLES

The main elements of a chronic disease management programme can be put in place using the same process, no

> **Box 16.1** Conditions suitable for a chronic disease management approach
>
> *Conditions include:*
>
> - asthma
> - diabetes
> - coronary heart disease
> - epilepsy
> - hypothyroidism
> - rheumatoid arthritis
> - osteoporosis
> - stress.

matter which condition is the subject of the programme, and whether the programme is based in general practice or in the community nursing services. The following guidelines can be applied to an asthma clinic, follow-up appointments for people with epilepsy, or women taking hormone replacement therapy, or any other long-term monitoring programme.

SETTING UP THE REGISTER

Before planning a programme, and throughout its implementation, it is important to find out:

- how many people in the surgery, or caseload, or area, have the condition
- who they are.

Numbers affected can initially be estimated from national prevalence figures. Asthma is thought to affect at least 10% of children: so a surgery with 500 children registered should have at least 50 children with asthma. Diabetes affects 1–2% of the population, and similar figures can be found for other chronic conditions. The number of people with a condition in one surgery, caseload or area will not match the expected prevalence exactly, but the figure can act as a guide to whether the proportion of people identified is comprehensive or not.

There are a number of ways in which the individual patients in the practice population, or on a caseload, who have a particular condition, can be traced:

- by searching the practice computer for appropriate disease codes assigned to patient records, e.g. all patients coded with diabetes mellitus
- by searching repeat prescribing records for appropriate drugs which indicate the condition, e.g. all forms of hormone replacement therapy

- by checking practice referral records, e.g. to find all people with coronary heart disease referred to a cardiovascular surgeon
- by asking professional colleagues and administrative staff for their knowledge of people with a particular condition
- by advertising through posters in a surgery or clinic, or by word of mouth, that a register is being set up, and asking patients to refer themselves to the appropriate professional.

The register can be kept on computer, or manually using a card index system. It is useful both for practical purposes and for audit and reporting to record some demographic information about the individuals on the register. Commonly this includes:

- age or age group
- sex
- ethnicity
- date of diagnosis.

This information enables the person running the programme to see if certain groups are better or worse served by the programme. For example, it may become apparent that men with asthma are frequent non-attenders at the asthma clinic, or people who have had diabetes for more than 10 years tend to ask for more appointments at the diabetic clinic. The timing, content and availability of the clinics may need to be reviewed as a result.

 Disease registers need to be continuously updated as people join or leave a caseload or area, and new patients are diagnosed.

ESTABLISHING A CALL AND RECALL SYSTEM

The purpose of a call and recall system is:

- to give people the opportunity to benefit from the chronic disease management programme, by letting them know when and how they can be seen
- to try to ensure that monitoring of the condition takes place at the most effective intervals, by giving people specific dates or intervals for follow-up appointments or visits
- to minimize the number of people who 'slip through the net' of monitoring and follow-up, and suffer unnecessary illness or complications as a result.

Call and recall systems, which send out invitations to relevant people to attend clinics or appointments, or to arrange a visit with a nurse, can be computer-run or manual. Some people are more likely to respond to and keep appointments if a letter is personalized, or signed by a professional, rather than generated automatically by a computer. In either case the letter will be most effective if it is:

- informative not directive
- specific not general
- encouraging not threatening.

> **!** Letters or invitation cards should be sent in envelopes so that the content is not apparent from the outside, in order to maintain patient confidentiality.

If people do not respond to a letter, and it is felt to be important for their health that they are seen in a chronic disease management programme, they can be contacted directly by telephone or visit. This has to be undertaken sensitively, and with care to maintain confidentiality about a patient's diagnosis and condition. Messages about clinics or appointments should not be left with relatives.

> **!** Remember that people have a right to choose how they care for their health, and the professional's role is to provide information and opportunities to enable them to make their choices.

PATIENT EDUCATION AND CONTINUING EDUCATION

Giving people opportunities to learn about their condition, its treatment and management, has two benefits:

- It increases their motivation to accept and comply with treatment.
- It fosters their independence and responsibility for their own care.

Educating patients consists of more than simply giving information. It also involves checking regularly:

- how much a person already knows
- how much they want to know

- what terms and ideas they are familiar with
- how much information they can accept at one time.

People vary in the extent to which they want to be in control of their condition, from those who want to know as much or more than the professionals, and decide their own programme of treatment, to those who would rather leave all decisions in the hands of others. Individuals may also want different types or depth of information at different stages of their condition or of their life. It is important that the nurse keeps checking that the patient is getting what they want. There are many resources available to help in patient education:

- Booklets, leaflets, videos, audio tapes and other sources of information can be offered to give factual information, or to present other patients' experiences which may be helpful.
- Devices such as placebo inhalers and dummy pill packets can be useful in teaching techniques to patients, and for allowing patients to practise themselves.

Sources for obtaining these resources are shown in Box 16.2.

Box 16.2 Obtaining resources for patient education

Sources of leaflets, videos, audiotapes:

- health education authority
- appropriate charities and societies (e.g. Royal National Institute for the Blind, British Diabetic Association)
- pharmaceutical companies making related drugs or products
- local hospital Trust departments
- other surgeries' resource libraries
- local primary care audit group resource library
- some computer software packages.

! It is very important that nurses demonstrating the use of devices to patients are able to do so correctly. Always check and practise before teaching patients.

PROTOCOLS FOR CLINICAL PROCEDURES

The clinical and other procedures to be carried out when a patient attends a chronic disease management consultation are the core of the programme. The key characteristics of the protocol are:

- It is specific to the practice or people involved.
- It is a working document.
- It is reviewed regularly.

Writing a protocol is not difficult, and often it is not necessary to start from scratch. There are many sample protocols available for asthma, diabetes, hypertension, epilepsy and other clinics. Sources are shown in Box 16.3. These samples can be adapted so that they are specific to the circumstances of the practice, or the nurses who will use them. There are also many evidence-based, 'best practice' guidelines produced by nationally credible expert groups, covering issues such as levels of glycaemia requiring referral or action, or 'step-wise' treatment in asthma, which can be adopted and incorporated into a local protocol. This part of the protocol becomes, in effect, an agreement that the surgery or team will all follow one set of credible guidelines.

Box 16.3   Sources of sample protocols

- practice nursing textbooks
- practice nurse support groups
- local primary care audit group resource library
- other surgeries
- appropriate hospital departments.

In producing a protocol for a clinic or service, it is essential that:

- Everyone who will use the protocol is involved in writing or adapting it.
- It reflects the real situation in which it will be used.
- It is agreed by everyone who will use it.

Practice nurses involved in producing surgery protocols should be able to involve themselves and the GP, as few people are involved. However, it is unlikely that all district nurses, health visitors and other Trust nurses will be able to be directly involved if a Trust-wide protocol is being produced, for example, for the treatment of leg ulcers. Representatives of the nursing groups will probably be involved, and other nurses must ensure that they contact their representative, review the work in progress and offer constructive comments to be conveyed to the working group.

The content of a protocol can be the same no matter which condition or disease management programme it refers to. Box 16.4 gives a generic protocol framework which could be followed.

The advantages of a realistic, working protocol for a chronic disease management programme are:

• All professionals involved give the same service to patients, on each occasion.
• All patients have equal access to information, investigation and referral.
• The service is based on 'best practice' guidelines, rather than individual practice.
• A nurse 'filling in' on a clinic or consultations for an absent colleague knows exactly what is usually done at a clinic or consultation.

Box 16.4 Suggested content of a chronic disease management protocol

• aim/objectives of management
• staff involved in managing disease and their qualifications/updating needs
• resources required for management (e.g. peak flow meters for asthma, glucometer for diabetes)
• measurements/procedures to be undertaken during the consultation
• information/education to be offered during the consultation
• recall intervals for patients
• method of audit of service.

⚠ Protocols should be signed and dated by the practitioners (or their representatives) involved in their production.

REFERRAL ARRANGEMENTS

This element of the programme covers two different situations:

• referral from the nurse back to the patient's GP
• referral from the primary health care team to secondary care.

The first is essential in a nurse-led chronic disease management programme. Guidelines used in the protocol will usually indicate at what level of blood pressure, glycaemia, peak expiratory flow rate or other parameter treatment needs to be started or reviewed. This is usually the point at which the patient needs to be referred back to the GP, or the GP needs to be informed, so that appropriate changes to treatment can be made.

> **!** Nurse prescribing is still a very limited activity, and nurses should ensure that they do not imply to patients that they can 'prescribe' treatment for chronic diseases, even though they are involved in explaining, demonstrating, administering and monitoring treatment.

Other points for referral back to the GP from a nurse-run programme are:

- when the patient is not responding to treatment in the expected way (e.g. an asthmatic still coughing at night) – this needs to be defined in the protocol
- after a period of time defined in the protocol (e.g. hypertensive patients to be reviewed by the GP at least once a year)
- when the patient needs an investigation which is beyond the nurse's competence (e.g. annual fundoscopy for people with diabetes)
- at any other time when the nurse does not feel competent to deal with the patient's condition or answer the patient's questions.

It is often difficult for a nurse who has been running a chronic disease management programme, and has the confidence and respect of the patients, to refer a patient back to the GP. However, it is essential for patient safety and professional accountability that such referrals are made. They can be treated as an opportunity for the nurse to learn and develop skills, rather than a failure or admission of fallibility.

> **!** The Code of Professional Conduct states: 'you must acknowledge any limitations in your knowledge and competence and decline any duties or responsibilities unless able to perform them in a safe and skilled manner'.

Referral from the primary health care team to secondary care often depends on individual GPs' preferences and clinical interests. Many districts have 'shared care' guidelines, drawn up by discussion between secondary care consultants and GPs, which set out when referrals will be made and accepted for different conditions. These can be referred to in the protocol, if there is agreement that they will be used by all GPs in a practice.

APPROPRIATE PERSONNEL AND TRAINING

The Code of Professional Conduct and the Scope of Professional Practice documents make it clear that nurses, midwives and health visitors must ensure that they act always within the limitations of their knowledge and competence. The management of a chronic disease requires a detailed knowledge and understanding of the condition, the treatments and drugs used to manage the condition, and the possible long-term consequences of the condition. Nurses involved in chronic disease management programmes need to ensure that they have this knowledge before taking on this responsibility. There are several ways that additional knowledge and competence can be gained:

- by undertaking a recognized course (see Box 16.5)
- by accessing appropriate modules of other courses
- by accessing appropriate skills-based training, and pursuing private study to gain the appropriate knowledge
- by finding in-house or informal training opportunities (in other surgeries or clinics, in outpatient sessions)
- by a combination of these methods.

Box 16.5 Recognized courses for chronic disease management

- ENB 285 Continuing care of the Dying Patient and the Family
- ENB A57 Nursing management of the client with continence care needs
- ENB N80 Chronic disease management for nurses
- ENB N83 Asthma management in acute and primary settings
- ENB N97 Diabetes nursing in the primary health care setting
- Diploma in Asthma Management, National Asthma Training Centre, Stratford-upon-Avon

---

! All registered nurses are professionally accountable for their own practice and need to be sure that they are competent in order to practise safely. Informal or in-house training may not involve an assessment of competence.

RECORD KEEPING

Complete and accurate records are essential to good patient care. They allow communication between professionals, and demonstrate the process of assessment and care of the patient. Good records are particularly effective in chronic disease management, when the patient may see a large number of different professionals over a long period of time. Records of chronic disease management consultations can be made in one or more of four places:

- the patient's GP notes, kept in the surgery
- the nursing records used by district nurses and other Trust nurses, and kept either by the nurse or in the patient's home
- on specially-designed cards specific to the condition (e.g. asthma, diabetes or menopause), kept in the surgery as part of the disease register
- on patient-held records.

The advantages and disadvantages of each form of record is shown in Table 16.1.

Whichever sort of records are kept, they fulfil several important functions. Specifically, they:

- provide information about the patient's condition and care
- provide a record of problems and actions taken to remedy them
- provide evidence of care required and delivered
- record physical, social and psychological factors affecting the patient
- support standard-setting and audit
- provide a baseline against which to monitor change.

Some basic guidelines, set out by the UKCC in its 'Standards for Records and Record-keeping', apply to all records, including those concerned with chronic disease management. All records should:

- be made as soon as possible after the events
- identify factors which put the patient, or standards of care, at risk
- provide evidence when there is need of special knowledge and skills
- help patients to be involved in their care
- protect staff against complaints
- be written in terms that the patient will understand.

Table 16.1
Advantages and disadvantages of different forms of record keeping for chronic diseases

	Advantages	Disadvantages
GP records	Contain complete history Cover all patient's conditions Easily accessible within surgery	Not available in patient's home Limited space for recording detail GPs may not want nurses to use Patient does not have easy access
Community nurse records (in patient's home)	Available to all visiting professionals to use Patient has access Space for recording detail Pre-printed with outline plan of care	Not available to nurses based in surgeries May be lost or defaced
Disease-specific record cards	Contain prompts for specific information Can incorporate self-management plan Keep all information on condition in one place Easy to file or carry	Deal with one condition in isolation Limit amount of information recorded
Patient-held records	Encourage patients to share responsibility for care Patients have access to information Contain educational as well as clinical information Can be available to all professionals wherever seen	Occasionally lost or defaced Not available unless produced by patient Usually not complete record of all conditions

⚠ Records should be legible, indelible, unambiguous, signed or initialled, and accurate in relation to date and time.

Practical points

• Make alterations only by scoring out with a single line, then initialling and dating the correct entry.

> ⚠️ **Do not use liquid paper to cover entries, and do not remove any part of the record to remove incorrect entries.**

• Avoid using pencil (which can be erased) or blue ink (which does not photocopy well).
• If initials rather than signatures are used, ensure that there are arrangements for identifying people from their initials.

AUDIT

> ⚠️ **Carrying out audit of the asthma and diabetic chronic disease management (CDM) programmes is a requirement for GPs claiming the CDM payment from their health authority.**

All chronic disease management programmes benefit from regular audit to see if standards of care are being maintained or improving. Since such programmes last for years, there is a real opportunity to improve the care of individual patients over time, and to track any improvements in patients' condition or outcome as a result of improved monitoring and care.

Different types of audit can be applied to a CDM programme:

• Critical event audit can be used to look at one particular event, good or bad, affecting a patient, and to learn something from it which can inform the care of other similar patients.
• Criteria-based audit can be used to measure the performance of a primary care team in managing the disease against local or national guidelines, then changes can be made to make it more likely that guidelines will be met or further exceeded.

The role of the nurse in audit should not be just data collecting, or data analysis. Interpretation of the findings, and making recommendations about and implementing changes, are central to the nurse's role as advocate for the patient.

SUMMARY

Most nurses in primary care are involved in the management of chronic diseases. An organized approach, using the guidelines set out for GPs' asthma and diabetes programmes, can be applied to any chronic condition. Nurses must ensure that they have adequate training and updating to be competent in monitoring complex and potentially damaging diseases.

Further reading

Hillson R 1996 Practical diabetes care. Oxford Medical Publications, Oxford

Kendrick M, Luker KA (eds) 1995 Clinical nursing practice in the community. Blackwell Science, Oxford

NHF 1995 Preventing coronary heart disease in primary care–the way forward. National Heart Forum, London

UKCC 1992a Code of professional conduct. UKCC, London

UKCC 1992b The scope of professional practice. UKCC, London

UKCC 1993 Standards for records and record keeping, UKCC, London

Health screening and assessment

The assessment of health and screening for disease is a common thread in many community nurses' work. For example:

• Midwives assess the health of pregnant women as well as monitoring the progress of the pregnancy.
• Health visitors screen young children for development problems, hearing and vision loss.
• School nurses screen school-age children for physical and mental health problems.
• Practice nurses, district nurses and sometimes other members of the team assess the health of elderly people.

There are many other examples of this area of practice, some of which are shown in Table 17.1. Such preventive and diagnostic activity affects most people at some stage in their lives, even if they remain entirely healthy. It is therefore an important interface between the vast majority of the public and the health service.

The fact that many people are, or believe themselves to be, in good health when they attend for health checks or

Table 17.1
Examples of screening and health assessment carried out in primary care

Type	Target group	Professionals usually involved
General health screening	All adults	Practice nurses, district nurses, health visitors, occupational health nurses
Child health surveillance	Children 0–5 years	GPs, health visitors
Diabetic eye screening	Diabetics	GPs, opticians
Diabetic foot screening	Diabetics	GPs, practice nurses, district nurses, chiropodists
HIV screening	Any individual on request	Some GPs, GUM depts
Rubella antibody screening	Pregnant women, women planning pregnancy	GPs, practice nurses, midwives

screening is an important factor in the relationship between the nurse and the individual. The person attending may be:

- convinced he is healthy, only to be told by the nurse that that may not be the case
- convinced she has a health problem, only to be told that there is no evidence of it
- resentful of the implication that he might be less than healthy
- afraid that something abnormal will be found
- irritated that 'the system' tracks her even when she doesn't initiate contact.

Of course many people treat health checks and screening tests as mundane chores. But it is worth remembering that this is not necessarily the case and an individual attending for a health check needs to be treated with the same degree of care and attention as a person attending for treatment of an illness.

 Remember that the identification of a previously unknown problem may have serious implications for the individual in terms of lifestyle (e.g. driving, occupation), need for treatment, insurance and even life expectancy.

DEFINITIONS

For the purposes of this chapter, 'screening' refers to activities designed to establish the presence or absence of a particular condition or marker for a condition. Examples would be taking a cervical smear to look for precancerous cells in the cervix, or measuring blood pressure to find out if a person is hypertensive. 'Health assessment' involves a range of different measurements, tests and enquiries, designed to uncover a wider picture of a person's health and wellbeing. Box 17.1 shows examples in each of these categories.

Many activities carried out by nurses in primary care combine elements of screening and health assessment in one meeting with a patient or client. A health visitor may 'screen' a child for hearing problems using a particular test, but may also use the occasion to make a much broader assessment of the child's health and development. These activities can also be divided into 'universal' or 'targeted' screening or assessment. Universal screening is carried out on a whole, defined population: for example, neonatal screening for phenylketonuria is universal, because all babies are tested for the condition. Targeted screening is aimed at a part of the

Box 17.1 Examples of screening and health assessment

Screening:
- cervical cytology
- mammography
- HIV testing
- audiometry
- rubella screening.

Assessment:
- well-man checks
- insurance 'medicals'
- teenage health clinics
- antenatal care
- pre-conceptual care.

population, or an individual, who may be at greater risk. Screening for some genetic disorders falls into this category, as screening will only be carried out in families known to be affected.

REASONS FOR SCREENING OR HEALTH ASSESSMENT

Screening and health assessment can be undertaken for a range of reasons, but there are common factors in this work, whoever carries it out.

In practical terms, there are six principal reasons for undertaking screening or health assessment:

- It is a contractual requirement.
- It is national or district policy.
- It is local protocol.
- It is good practice.
- It is indicated clinically.
- It is requested by the individual.

Some examples of screening and assessment in each of these categories are shown in Table 17.2.

COMMON FACTORS IN SCREENING AND HEALTH ASSESSMENT

Whatever kind of screening or health assessment is being carried out, and for whatever reason, there are a number of common factors to all such encounters.

Table 17.2
Examples of different reasons for undertaking screening or health assessments

Reason	Type of screening/assessment
Contractual requirement (for GPs)	Over-75-years assessment New-patient health assessment
National/district policy	Neonatal screening for phenylketonuria Cervical cancer screening Child health surveillance
Good practice	Screening for therapeutic drug plasma levels, e.g. thyroxine, antiepileptic drugs
Clinically indicated	Screening for toxoplasmosis in pregnant woman with symptoms HIV screening Screening for iron deficiency anaemia
Requested by individual	Well-woman assessment 'Medical' for insurance purposes

Consent

The consent of the individual must always be obtained for invasive procedures to be undertaken, such as blood tests or examinations. It is good practice to ask permission for non-invasive aspects of the assessment too. When sensitive questions are to be asked, it is useful to signal this and check that the individual is agreeable. For example: 'Now I need to ask you about your previous pregnancies: is this okay?'

> ⚠ Some screening tests may require the written consent of the person undergoing the test; always check with local surgery or Trust protocols whether this is the case, and if so, who should obtain the consent.

Protocol

A protocol or procedure for the assessment or screening test should be available to any nurse undertaking it. This sets out what tests or examinations are to be undertaken, or what questions are to be asked. It should also indicate when particular findings such as raised blood pressure warrant referral to another member of the team, or trigger another test. These protocols can be very important in guiding the nurse about what not to do, as well as what to do. For example, many practice nurses used to undertake breast examinations during well-women clinics. This is not now recommended practice and protocols for well-woman clinics should reflect this change.

Training and preparation

The nurse carrying out the assessment or screening must have sufficient training and preparation for the task. Competence in the technical tasks involved – such as venepuncture or taking a cervical smear – is not enough. The person undergoing screening will need information about the condition screened for, and the nature and interpretation of tests and examinations involved. They may also ask about the prevalence of the condition, and the consequences of positive findings. It is important that they can be given sufficient, accurate information to enable them to give informed consent to the procedures, and to alleviate as far as possible the concerns they may have about the screening.

> ⚠ **Preparation does not necessarily have to consist of a training course. Reading, working with colleagues, private study or visits to other screening units can also help.**

Resources

Resources, both for carrying out tests and observations, and for teaching people about them, should be available when and where the screening or assessment is taking place. Equipment needs to be appropriate, well maintained and accurate, if results of observations and examinations are to be used to diagnose conditions and indicate the need for treatment. For example, simple checks on an instrument such as a sphygmomanometer (see Box 17.2) can indicate whether the reading is likely to be accurate, and ensure that a lifelong diagnosis of hypertension is not made in error. Instruments used on more than one patient, such as vaginal speculae used in taking cervical smears, must be sterilized between use, and the mechanism for storage, cleaning and sterilization should be known to the nurse before the instrument is used.

> **Box 17.2** Checking a mercury sphygmomanometer
>
> Ensure that:
>
> • The equipment has been serviced within the last 6 months.
> • The mercury is at zero before measurement begins.
> • The column is upright at a right angle to the base.
> • The glass is clean.
> • The tubing is not perished.
> • The valve does not leak air.
> • The column of mercury can be viewed at eye level during use.

> ⚠ **The nurses' Code of Conduct requires that 'no action or omission on your part, or within your sphere of responsibility, is detrimental to the interests, condition or safety of patients'.**

Using resources in people's homes can present particular problems. To minimize the chance of inaccurate readings:

• Place portable scales for measuring weight on hard surfaces, not carpet.
• Ensure that sphygmomanometers rest in an upright, not tilted, position, and that the zero marking on the mercury column is level with the heart.
• Check that containers to be used for urine samples are clean and free from contaminants.

Consistency

Consistency of approach and information amongst the primary health care team are very important. Each member of the team should know:

• which screening or assessment tests are undertaken by which members of the team at what intervals
• which tests are not undertaken by the team, and why
• how long different test results take to return from the laboratory
• what is the surgery or clinic procedure for patients to obtain the results of tests which have been sent away for analysis
• who is responsible for ensuring maintenance and checking of equipment.

Record keeping

Record keeping is as important to screening and assessment activities as it is to patient care during illness or treatment. The UKCC 'Standards for Records and Record-Keeping' (1993) require records to contain 'all significant consultations, assessments, observations, decisions, interventions and outcomes'. People will sometimes ask for a 'quick check' of their blood pressure, or urine, or other factor, just for reassurance. It is important that these very informal forms of screening or assessment are recorded in the person's record in the same way as a planned consultation.

 A negative finding may be as significant as a positive one, and should always be recorded.

There may be occasions when an individual requests that a screening test is not recorded in their record: for example, a pregnancy test, or a test for sexually transmitted disease. Rather than make individual decisions, nurses should ensure that they follow the surgery or trust protocol on these issues. This is one reason why it is important to know the test or screening protocol in advance.

EXAMPLES OF SCREENING PROGRAMMES

NEW-PATIENT CHECKS

The GP Contract of 1990 introduced a new requirement for GPs to offer a health assessment to anyone between the ages of 5 and 74 years who joined their list. This universal health assessment has become known as the 'new-patient check'. These health checks are usually carried out by the practice nurse, and consist of:

- a review of the individual's medical history
- recording of any current medical problems
- recording of any medicines taken regularly
- recording of any allergies or adverse reactions to medicines or other substances
- review of immunization and screening history
- measurement of height and weight, calculation of body mass index, measurement of blood pressure, routine urinalysis
- administration of any vaccines required
- other screening tests, such as cholesterol or cervical smear, as appropriate.

The new-patient check is also an opportunity for health promotion, targeted specifically at the individual and family.

The advantages of new-patient screening are that information is gathered systematically, often in advance of the patient's medical record being sent on from his/her previous doctor. This prevents delay if treatment, repeat prescriptions or new referrals to secondary care are required.

OVER-75 CHECKS

Another element of the GP's Terms of Service is the requirement to offer a health check, at home, to all patients on their list who are over the age of 75 years. This check has to include, where appropriate:

- assessment of physical condition, including continence
- assessment of mental condition
- assessment of sensory functions (e.g. vision and hearing)
- assessment of mobility
- recording of current medication
- assessment of social and home environment.

The check is often carried out by a member of the practice's primary health care team, such as the practice nurse, district nurse or health visitor, rather than by the GP.

> **!** It is essential that such checks are only carried out by nurses who are trained and competent to do so.

Practice protocols for the assessment of the physical health, included in the over-75 check, usually involve:

- measurement of blood pressure
- calculation of body mass index
- urinalysis
- review of immunization status (e.g. against tetanus, and hepatitis A for frequent travellers), with vaccination offered as necessary
- recording of risk factors such as high levels of alcohol consumption and smoking.

In practice, some people decline the over-75 check when offered, and others will visit the surgery rather than be visited at home.

The advantages of this check are that some physical, mental or social problems can be detected early, and treatment or assistance offered. The check also offers the opportunity for an annual review of medication, which can be complex and even dangerous when many different drugs are involved.

> ⚠️ **A local pharmacist is sometimes contracted to review the medication of elderly patients as part of their over-75 check: a pharmacist is appropriately qualified to advise on possible drug interactions, and on reducing polypharmacy.**

CHILD HEALTH SURVEILLANCE

This is probably one of the best-known forms of universal screening. It is a programme of care which aims to prevent illness and promote good health and development for all children. The content of the current programme was set out in a consensus report (the Hall Report) by the Joint Working Party on Child Health Surveillance, which consisted of paediatricians, GPs, health visitors and nurses. The specific aims of the programme are shown in Box 17.3.

While the child health surveillance programme currently covers all children, the 'inverse care law' may apply, and families whose children have the most needs are sometimes the least likely to attend for appointment, or ask for help and support. The families which have been suggested as priority groups are:

- very young or unsupported parents
- parents of limited intelligence and education
- parents thought to be at particular risk of abusing their children

---

Box 17.3 Aims of the child health surveillance programme

The programme's aims are:

- the promotion of optimal health and development
- the prevention of illness, accidents and child abuse
- the recognition and, if possible, elimination of potential problems affecting development, behaviour and education
- the early detection of abnormality, in order to offer investigation and treatment.

From Hall et al (1994).

- parents who are socially isolated due to personality, psychiatric, linguistic or cultural factors
- families living in extreme poverty or temporary accommodation
- high-achieving parents with high personal standards for themselves (Hall et al 1994).

Whatever the social or other circumstances of the families involved, it is important that nurses and health visitors involved in child health surveillance avoid judgmental attitudes.

> ⚠ 'The role of the health professional is to be a friend and adviser of the parent(s) – the relationship should be established on equal terms, rather than with the professional in the dominant role' (Hall et al 1994).

In some areas of the country there are moves to restrict child health surveillance activities, especially those of Trust-based staff such as health visitors, to targeted 'high risk' families, rather than continuing with a universal programme. The advantage of freeing time to spend with families who clearly have difficulties has to be weighed against the disadvantages of failing to identify needs at an early stage, when intervention might prevent or ameliorate a problem. This issue will probably continue to be debated for some time.

GENERAL PRACTITIONERS AND CHILD HEALTH SURVEILLANCE

The 1990 GP Contract allowed GPs to register with their local Family Health Services Authority (now Health Authority) to provide child health surveillance programmes to under 5 year olds, and to receive a supplementary fee for each child for whom they provide this service. A GP has to have completed an approved training course to be eligible to provide child surveillance. In practice the surveillance programme is usually provided by a multidisciplinary team including the GP and health visitor, as well as the practice nurse for some aspects such as immunization.

> ⚠ Each primary health care team should have an agreed protocol for the child health surveillance programme, so that all members are clear about their contribution.

The programme of review of a child's health usually follows the timetable shown in Box 17.4. Undertaking the assessments and examinations involved, and interpreting the overall picture of the child's health and development, requires specialist training such as that of the health visitor. It should not be undertaken by nurses who have not acquired the necessary skills.

Box 17.4 The child health surveillance programme

Check includes the following.

8 weeks:
- review of progress with parents
- general examination, including for jaundice, any abnormal physical features, all systems, head circumference
- assessment of development, physical and social
- test for congenital dislocation of the hip
- check for congenital cataract
- check test results (PKU, thyroid, sickle cell if done).

6–9 months:
- review of progress with parents
- assessment of development, physical and social
- check for hip stability
- 'distraction test' for hearing
- physical examination including heart, and measurement of length, weight, head circumference.

18–24 months:
- review of progress with parents
- assessment of development, including communication, mobility, behaviour
- measurement of height.

3–5 years:
- review of progress with parents
- assessment of mobility, language, social development
- general physical check, including height
- any other clinically indicated tests.

From Hall et al (1994).

PARENT-HELD RECORDS

In many parts of the country, parents are given a 'personal child health record' (PCHR) soon after the birth of their child. The use of PCHRs is encouraged by the Department of Health, and there is national agreement about the format and content, although there may be minor local variations. The advantages of a PHCR are:

• It encourages the parents to contribute to their child's health records.
• It encourages partnership between parents and professionals, as parents can see what health professionals have recorded about their child's health and development.
• It means that all pertinent information about a child's health and development is contained in one record which can be taken to appointments with any professional.
• It provides written health advice and information for parents.

> ⚠ It is essential that health professionals always use the PCHR when it is available, and remind parents to bring it to appointments.

In districts where the PCHR is in use, it is usually regarded as the main record, and the information recorded in it is not duplicated in separate community-nursing or health-visiting notes. This generally applies even when there is a problem with a child's care or development, including when child abuse is suspected.

> ⚠ Under current legislation, parents can demand to see any record kept about them or their children, so keeping information in a separate record from the PCHR will not 'protect' it from their knowledge.

Nurses working for a Trust should always check and follow the trust's own policy on record keeping.

SUMMARY

Health screening and assessment is a common activity for nurses in primary care. It should always be based on partnership and openness with the person being screened, and the nurse should be aware of the implications for the individual of identifying possible health risks or problems. Some forms of screening (e.g. of mental health, or of children's development) require specialist training, and should only be undertaken by appropriately trained and/or qualified personnel. The use of patient or parent-held records, when screening takes place over a long period of time, both encourages openness and sharing of information, and ensures that all information is kept in one place for easy reference.

References

Hall D, Hill P, Elliman D 1994 The child health surveillance handbook, 2nd edn. Radcliffe Medical Press, Oxford

UKCC 1993 Standards for records and record-keeping. UKCC, London

Further reading

Idris Williams E 1995 Caring for older peole in the community, 3rd edn. Radcliffe Medical Press, Oxford

RCN 1991 Guidelines for assessment of elderly people. Royal College of Nursing, London

18

Child protection

The physical, sexual or other abuse of children is an issue of concern to all health professionals. Some community nurses – in particular health visitors and school nurses – have a role in the formal child protection procedures which exist in every health district. Other community nurses, who do not have a formal role, still have responsibilities in child protection: principally in recognizing and reporting suspected abuse. It is an area of practice which frequently worries practitioners. However, it is also an area in which clear procedures and protocols exist, and multi-agency cooperation is generally very well developed. Provided individual nurses are aware of local procedures, and of the limits of their own responsibility, they should be able to practise confidently.

BACKGROUND

Local authority child protection registers record four types of abuse:

- neglect
- physical injury
- sexual abuse
- emotional abuse.

A child's name can be placed on the register by a child protection conference if it has suffered, or is thought likely to suffer, 'significant harm' from one or more identifiable incidents in any of these categories. The child protection register is maintained by local social services departments, and is a confidential document, although health professionals working with a child who need to know if the child's name is on a register can apply for access to the register. Every child whose name is on the child protection register will have an assigned 'key worker', and an agreed protection plan aimed at preventing further abuse or risk to the child.

A Department of Health study of child abuse inquiry reports (DoH 1991), and a study of child abuse and neglect deaths (Greenland 1988), identified some common factors in families in which abuse had taken place. These included:

- parental history of unstable, damaging or violent adult relationships
- parental violence outside the family
- deaths of other children within the family
- parents abused or neglected as children
- parents aged 20 or less at birth of first child
- single, separated or divorced parent
- partner not biological parent
- alcohol or drug abuse
- social isolation

- poverty
- poor housing/frequent house moves.

> ⚠ **The absence of all these factors does not mean that abuse has not occurred: child abuse could occur in any family in any circumstances.**

Signs of physical abuse can include:

- bruises, often at various stages of healing
- burns
- bite marks
- fractures
- black eyes
- pain around the genital area (in sexual abuse).

> ⚠ **These injuries may also occur accidentally, and distinguishing non-accidental injuries is a task for specialists with training and experience.**

THE CHILDREN ACT 1989

The principal legislation concerning the welfare of children is The Children Act 1989. It brings together the law relating to individuals and the law relating to public bodies such as health authorities and local authorities. The Act is designed to promote the interests of the child, and balances family autonomy against the rights of children.

The Children Act has a number of central principles, including:

- The welfare of the child is the paramount consideration in most court proceedings.
- Wherever possible, children should be brought up and cared for within their own families.
- Children should be safe and be protected by effective intervention if they are in danger – but this should be open to challenge by parents in the courts.
- Children should be kept informed about what happens to them, and should participate when decisions are made about their future if they are of an age and understanding to do so.
- Parents continue to have parental responsibility for their children even when their children are no longer living with them.

The Children Act also sets out a number of court orders which may be applied to children:

- A care order places the child in the care of the local authority and gives the authority shared parental responsibility, with the parents, for the child; it will only be made if the court believes that a child is suffering or likely to suffer significant harm through lack of adequate parental care or control.
- A supervision order puts the child under the supervision of a local authority or probation officer, without giving the authority or officer any parental responsibility.
- A child assessment order (under section 43) is made in situations where there is evidence that a child is suffering or is likely to suffer significant harm but is not at immediate risk, and the applicant believes that a medical or psychiatric assessment is required, but the child's parents are unwilling to cooperate. The order lasts a maximum of 7 days and the court decides the extent and type of the assessment.
- An emergency protection order (under sections 44 and 45) is made in urgent cases when the child's safety is immediately threatened; it lasts for 8 days, with one extension of 7 days possible, and gives the applicant (usually the local authority or the NSPCC) parental responsibility for the child insofar as necessary to safeguard and promote the welfare of the child.

> **!** Specialized training in this area of practice is essential for community nurses who will be involved in carrying out assessments or making reports for court proceedings.

THE AREA CHILD PROTECTION COMMITTEE (ACPC)

Every district has an ACPC which coordinates inter-agency child protection procedures. Membership of the ACPC is agreed locally, and comprises senior representatives from all agencies involved with the protection of children. These usually include:

- social services
- health authorities
- NHS trusts
- education authorities
- police and probation agencies
- local authority legal advisers.

Community nurses are represented on the ACPC by the senior manager with responsibility for community services, or for child protection, from their employing trust. Practice nurses can also contact this individual for information about local child protection policies, procedures and training.

> ⚠ **All community nurses should ensure that they know who is the local person with responsibility for child protection.**

CHILD PROTECTION CONFERENCES

The child protection conference, often referred to as the 'case conference', is the central part of the child protection process. It can only be convened by social services or the NSPCC, although it may be requested by other professionals. After an initial referral, often from the child's GP or health visitor, a social worker will visit the family, usually within 24 hours, to assess whether a child protection conference should be called. If a conference does take place, representatives from all agencies working directly with the child will be invited to attend to discuss whether it is necessary to enter the child onto the child protection register, and what can be done to protect the child from harm or risk in future. Parents are usually invited to at least part of the meeting, and the child may also be invited if they are old enough to understand.

> ⚠ **Procedures for meetings, record keeping and confidentiality will be set out in local trust protocols. Any nurse who might be involved in a conference should have attended training to ensure they are familiar with these protocols.**

If a child's name is placed on the child protection register, review conferences are held at least every 6 months. In the meantime a key social worker is appointed to carry out a more detailed assessment of the child and family, and to draw up a protection plan in consultation with other professionals.

ROLES OF COMMUNITY NURSES

Trust-employed health visitors and school nurses who may become involved in the formal processes of assessment, child protection conferences and protection plans will receive specialized training in these areas. They will also have access to the Trust's designated senior nurse for child protection, and may have specialist clinical supervision relating to child protection.

Other community nurses employed by Trusts, such as district nurses, midwives and community paediatric nurses, should also receive training in the recognition of possible child abuse and the procedures to follow for referral to appropriate professionals and agencies.

> **!** **Trust-employed nurses should ensure that they are familiar with and comply with Trust procedures related to child protection.**

Practice nurses who are directly employed by GPs are often isolated from the support and advice of more experienced managers. They should negotiate with their employers for the training necessary to enable them to identify possible child abuse. In the first instance they should always report suspicions to the child's GP or health visitor, who can make the necessary further investigations and referrals if appropriate.

> **!** **Practice nurses should ensure that there is a protocol in place for the specific actions to be taken in that practice if child abuse is suspected, and that it includes contact names and numbers (usually social services) for use in an emergency if the first-line of referral (GP or health visitor) is not available.**

Child protection is a complex and sensitive area of practice, and it is important that nurses do not try to take on too much responsibility. There are some general dos and don'ts for nurses in primary care who do not have a formal role in child protection. They are:

Do

- remember that the child's interests are paramount
- ensure that you have regular training and updating in the recognition of child abuse
- keep accurate, detailed records of any visible injury you are concerned about
- report any suspicions to the child's GP or health visitor as soon as possible
- know whom to contact for advice and support about child protection
- know and keep to Trust/practice protocols.

Don't

- carry out any examination beyond what you would normally include in the work you are undertaking with the child
- try to interview the child about the suspected injury or abuse
- try to confront or question parents
- defer referral for any reason.

SUMMARY

Child protection is a specialized and well-developed field. Those community nurses whose work includes specific responsibilities for child protection will have specialist training in the necessary assessment and other procedures. Other nurses need to be able to identify possible abuse and refer appropriately to other members of the primary health care team.

References

Department of Health 1991 Child abuse: a study of inquiry reports 1980–1989. HMSO, London

Greenland C 1988 Preventing child abuse and neglect deaths: an international study. Tavistock, London

Further reading

Department of Health 1991 Working together under the Children Act 1989–a guide to arrangements for interagency cooperation for the protection of children from abuse. HMSO, London

DoH 1996 The Children Act 1989: what every nurse, health visitor and midwife needs to know. Department of Health, London

HVA 1994 Protecting the child–an HVA guide to practice and procedures. Health Visitors' Association, London

19

Protection of other vulnerable groups

Children are possibly the most obvious, but not the only, vulnerable group in society. Other groups of individuals who may need additional protection include older people, the physically or mentally disabled, and those who are vulnerable to 'hidden' injury or abuse, such as 'domestic' violence.

Nurses working in primary care, visiting people in their own homes, or dealing with them regularly over long periods of time, are in a prime position to identify such vulnerable people, to help them to protect themselves and to spot signs of injury or abuse if it occurs. The difference between these forms of abuse and the abuse of children is that statutory procedures for dealing with these cases do not exist in the same clear form, and there are no district committees with the responsibility to oversee action. It is therefore even more important that nurses are aware of the possibility of abuse, and the actions they can take to prevent it, or deal with it if it occurs.

ELDER ABUSE

This can take a number of forms, some of which are not easy to identify. They include:

- physical abuse – including generally rough handling, such as squeezing and pushing as well as actual violence
- psychological abuse – including threats of violence, verbal abuse, frightening behaviour
- sexual abuse – in many forms, and of both men and women
- neglect – such as failure to ensure adequate food and heating is available, failure to seek medical help for a vulnerable person when it is needed, or failure to administer necessary medicines
- financial abuse – including taking money, pension or allowance books, or disposing of a person's assets without their consent.

People who are most vulnerable to such abuse are:

- the very elderly
- those with physical or mental health problems
- the more dependent elderly.

Elder abuse is usually carried out by a member of the person's family, or a carer (who may be an informal carer or a professional carer) who is in frequent contact with them. The abuser may be under considerable stress, and have health or financial difficulties themselves.

> ⚠ If, as a nurse, you have concerns about 'inappropriate behaviour' by another nurse you will need to report your concerns to the appropriate person or authority: usually your manager in the first instance.

Abuse may be suspected because of:

- visible bruising, scratches or other injuries; unexplained injuries
- repeated failure of carer to bring the person for appointments or blood tests
- repeated failure to request repeat prescriptions when they are due
- fearfulness or withdrawal by the elderly person
- repeated visits by an elderly person to a nurse without clear reasons
- complaints or reports from the elderly person.

> ⚠ **As with other forms of abuse, it can be difficult to decide whether a plausible explanation for possible signs of abuse is true. If in doubt, arrange for another nursing colleague or the person's GP to give an opinion.**

There are actions which can be initiated by the primary health care team to help to prevent the abuse of dependent elderly people. These are aimed at relieving the stress and isolation of carers, and maintaining vigilance and communication amongst members of the team.

To support the carers:

• Keep a register of people caring for elderly relatives, so that appropriate information and support can be targeted at them.
• Advertise carers' group meetings, telephone help lines and crisis services on surgery and health centre notice boards.
• Investigate all forms of respite provision – day care places, beds, holidays, night sitters, day sitters, lunch clubs, volunteer carers – so that usual carers can have at least an occasional break.
• Offer health checks or visits to carers, who are often older and may be in poor health themselves.
• Listen for and act on cues from carers who are becoming desperate.

To maintain vigilance in the team:

• Include reminders to check for signs of abuse in protocols for over-75-year health assessments, routine elderly visiting and family visits.
• Discuss any concerns as soon as they arise with other members of the team.
• Record concerns, and reasons for them, in patient records, and discuss with the patient's GP.
• Agree a protocol for referral of abuse to appropriate agencies (see Table 19.1), including who will action the referral, and how the rest of the team will be informed that such as referral has taken place, and kept up to date with developments.

Table 19.1 Where to report abuse of an elderly person	
Circumstances of abuse	*Report to*
Nursing home, hospice, residential home	Health Authority Nursing Homes Inspection Unit
Residential care	Local Authority Inspection Unit
NHS community hospital, clinic, day care centre	Trust which runs the facility
Client's home	Social Services community assessment team

> ⚠ **Reports of abuse cases of all kinds invariably highlight a lack of communication between professionals as a contributory factor to unchecked abuse.**

ABUSE IN THE HOME

Any adult may be abused in their own home, and abuse is usually carried out by a member of their family. Men as well as women may be victims, and children may abuse parents as well as adults abusing each other. People who are physically weaker or mentally impaired are more vulnerable to abuse of all kinds than others. Abuse of people with learning disabilities living in group homes or small institutions also falls into this category.

As with elderly people, abuse may be physical, psychological, financial or sexual in nature, or take the form of neglect.

As with elder abuse, the nurse's role includes:

- being alert for signs of abuse
- sharing concerns with colleagues so that a fuller assessment can be made
- maintaining full records of any signs observed or injuries treated
- identifying key resources such as help lines, support groups, statutory agencies and volunteer workers which can be offered to those in need of them
- maintaining systems for communication between members of the primary health care team and the GP.

AVOIDING PITFALLS

Dealing with suspicions of, or proven, abuse is a difficult area. Professional imperatives and values have to be applied alongside the requirements of trust procedures and of the law. A number of different agencies – social services, the police, solicitors and voluntary groups – may be involved as well as different NHS bodies and professionals. To minimize the chances of professional censure, a nurse dealing with any form of abuse at any stage, from suspicion to aftermath, should:

- seek the advice and involvement of a senior colleague, manager or GP, at an early stage
- ensure that they have adequate knowledge and skills in the relevant area, and refuse to take on tasks for which they do not have relevant knowledge and skills
- keep clear, objective and accurate records
- make use of all forms of professional support such as specialist groups, clinical supervision sessions and team meetings
- consult professional association representatives if there is any difficulty with obtaining adequate professional support locally.

To minimize both professional risk and personal stress, it is important *not* to:

- try to investigate claims or interview people
- be confrontational or accusatorial
- take on a case of abuse alone
- take sides in a family's or couple's disputes
- try to solve a problem yourself
- make unrealistic promises to a client.

CONFIDENTIALITY

The UKCC Code of Professional Conduct states that registered nurses must 'protect all confidential information concerning patients and clients obtained in the course of professional practice and make disclosures only with consent, where required by the order of a court or where you can justify disclosure in the wider public interest'. The UKCC's 'Guidelines for professional practice' define the public interest as 'the interests of an individual, groups of individuals or society as a whole', and covers:

- serious crime
- child abuse
- 'other activities which place others at serious risk'.

> ⚠️ **Sharing of information about clients between professionals who are or will be involved in the care of that client is part of normal professional practice.**

In dealing with abuse, however, it may be necessary to share information gained in the course of practice with people other than the health professionals caring for the client, such as social workers or the police. In this case, the breach of confidentiality has to be:

- with the client's permission, or
- in the public interest.

> ⚠️ **The advice and support of senior colleagues or managers should be sought in this situation.**

SUMMARY

Abuse can take many forms, and can affect people from any group in society. It is important that nurses have the resources, training, systems and support in place to work with clients in these situations. Professional advice and support, and a team approach, are essential to avoid professional and personal difficulties when working in this difficult area.

Further reading

Decalmer P, Glendenning F (eds) 1993 The mis-treatment of elderly people. Sage, London

Kingston P, Penhale B (eds) 1995 Family violence and the caring professions. Macmillan, London

UKCC 1992 Code of Professional Conduct. UKCC, London

UKCC 1996 Guidelines for professional practice. UKCC, London

SECTION 4

Treatment and care

20

Wound care

The presence of wounds, surgical or traumatic, is not confined to patients in hospital. Some nurses in primary care spend a large proportion of their time dealing with wounds. As wound treatments, and methods of dressing wounds, are subject to constant research and change, this is an area in which constant learning and updating are essential. Specific treatment regimes will not be discussed in this chapter for this reason.

There are four main types of wounds which fall into the community nurse's caseload:

- leg ulcers – mostly dealt with by district nurses and practice nurses
- surgical wounds – also dealt with by district nurses and practice nurses
- minor traumatic wounds – usually dealt with by practice nurses
- pressure sores – dealt with by district nurses and nurses working in nursing homes.

LEG ULCERS

Leg ulcers are 'areas of loss of skin below the knee on the leg or foot which take more than 6 weeks to heal' NHSCRD 1997). They may be arterial or venous (or mixed) in origin. Arterial ulcers develop as a result of arterial insufficiency caused by narrowing or obstruction of the arteries in the leg. The tissues ulcerate and die. While stopping smoking and increasing exercise may help to heal the ulcer, surgery is often necessary to restore an adequate blood supply to the lower leg. Most patients with an arterial ulcer will require referral to a vascular surgeon for assessment.

Venous ulcers are caused by a reduction in the efficiency of the back flow of blood from the lower leg to the heart. Such inefficiency can be caused by:

- immobility
- phlebitis
- deep vein thrombosis
- varicose veins
- leg injury.

Signs of venous hypertension caused by inadequate return include brown pigmentation of the skin on the lower leg, which is also harder than normal, and distended capillaries over the ankle region. The different presentations between venous and arterial ulcers are shown in Table 20.1.

Treatment of venous ulcers combines three elements:

- a dressing to encourage healing of the ulcer itself
- compression bandaging to assist venous return from the leg

Table 20.1
Different signs and symptoms from arterial and venous leg ulcers

Arterial ulcers	Venous ulcers
Skin shiny and hairless	Skin brown-stained
Pain on exercise, relieved by rest or hanging legs over edge of bed	Pain relieved by elevation and compression
Skin cool and pale	Skin warm
Absent or weak foot pulses	Strong foot pulses
Develop rapidly	Develop slowly
Usually small, deep, well defined	Usually larger, shallow, poorly defined edge

- attention to any lifestyle or medical factors which can be modified to increase the rate of healing and prevent recurrence (see below).

> ⚠ **Differentiation between venous, arterial and mixed aetiology ulcers (i.e. those with some arterial component) is vital, as the compression therapy used for venous ulcers is absolutely contraindicated for arterial ulcers.**

Differentiation requires a full assessment of both the individual and the ulcer. This assessment usually includes a measurement of the ankle brachial pressure index (ABPI) using a Doppler ultrasonograph.

> ⚠ **This assessment should be carried out by someone who has undertaken specific training in the use of the Doppler.**

SURGICAL WOUNDS

With the increase in day surgery and quicker discharge of surgical patients to their homes, even after major surgery, nurses in primary care see many more wounds at an earlier stage of healing than used to be the case. Surgical wounds are not necessarily incisions healing by primary intention (see below). Skin graft sites, for example, heal by secondary intention, and may require monitoring for a longer period of time.

The role of nurses in the community is usually

- to check for problems in the wound, e.g. infection, haematoma
- to remove sutures or other wound closures.

Mobile patients who have had relatively minor surgery may attend their GP's surgery to be seen by the practice nurse, while others are seen in their own homes by the district nurse.

WOUND INFECTION

 It is not good practice to take routine wound swabs in the absence of any clinical signs of infection.

Signs of infection in a wound are redness, pain, swelling, exudate of pus, and warmth at the wound site. Wound infections are usually treated by systemic antibiotics, as local antibiotics encourage the development of resistance in the infecting organisms.

 As nurse prescribers cannot prescribe antibiotics, these will always require referral to the patient's GP.

The removal of sutures or other skin closures is undertaken using the same techniques as in hospital settings. Hospital discharge letters or referral forms will usually indicate the day on which it is anticipated that sutures should be removed, but the wound should still be assessed by the nurse undertaking the procedure prior to the removal of closures.

MINOR TRAUMATIC WOUNDS

People may present to their doctor's surgery with a wide range of minor injuries. The commonest are

- burns and scalds
- cuts and abrasions
- foreign bodies.

BURNS AND SCALDS

Burns and scalds require immersion in cold water, or to be held under cold running water, as a first-aid measure. They can then be dressed with appropriate creams if prescribed. Pain from even superficial burns can be intense, and people should always be offered advice about suitable analgesics. Return appointments are advised, to check on the progress of healing, and that the burn has not become secondarily infected.

> ⚠ **Burns which are anything other than superficial, and superficial burns on the face, should always be seen by the GP or referred on after first-aid treatment so that the possibility of future scarring or contracture can be assessed.**

During later visits, there will be an opportunity to assess the background to the current injury, and the likelihood of a repeat injury. The individual may need advice about avoiding accidents in the home or at work, or, if confusion or dementia was a factor in the injury, further assessment of the individual and their circumstances will be necessary.

CUTS AND ABRASIONS

Cuts and abrasions which are presented to the practice nurse at a surgery may result from falls, bites, occupational injuries, accidents in the home, or assaults. Whatever the source, the priorities are

- assessment of the injury (which may also need the GP's opinion)
- cleaning and removal of any foreign bodies such as grit or glass
- suturing if required
- dressing of the injury
- pain relief
- assessment of immunization status (e.g. against tetanus: see Box 20.1).
- advice to the patient on care of the wound and dressing
- return appointment for reassessment of the injury.

If the injury is particularly painful because of its size, location or the amount of debris to be removed, it may be dealt with in the surgery as a minor operation requiring local anaesthesia (see Chapter 23).

Box 20.1 Wounds requiring tetanus immunization

'For immunised adults, who have received five doses [of tetanus vaccine] booster doses are not recommended, other than at the time of tetanus prone injury, since they have been shown to be unnecessary and can cause considerable local reactions.'

Tetanus prone wounds are:
• those sustained more than 6 hours before surgical treatment of wound or burn
• any wound or burn at any interval after injury that shows one or more of the following characteristics:
  – a significant degree of devitalized tissue
  – puncture type wound
  – contact with soil or manure likely to harbour tetanus organisms
  – clinical evidence of sepsis.

The recommended regimes of tetanus immunization, with either tetanus vaccine or tetanus immunoglobulin, are detailed in 'Immunisation against infectious disease', Department of Health, 1996.

From Department of Health (1996).

> **!** It is important that all dirt and foreign material is removed from wounds otherwise healing may be delayed and the cosmetic result can be worse.

A range of cleaning solutions, sutures and dressing materials are normally stocked in every surgery. These can be replaced by issuing the patient with a prescription after treatment, so that they can bring materials back to the surgery on their repeat visits.

> **!** Any individual who has sustained an injury from an assault or an accident which may result in an insurance or compensation claim (e.g. road accident or industrial accident) should have his/her injuries assessed and documented by a doctor.

Some GPs will always prescribe antibiotics after certain types of injury, e.g. human bites, or animal bites when there has been a delay in seeking treatment. Where this is the case, the importance of finishing the course of the antibiotic, and the possible side effects and interactions caused by antibiotics, should be clearly explained to the patient.

> ⚠️ **Some antibiotics cause nausea and vomiting, and so render the oral contraceptive pill less effective. Women who take the OCP should always be advised to use additional contraceptive protection if this is the case.**

FOREIGN BODIES

Foreign bodies may be present in almost any part of the body. They may be

- objects inserted by children into an ear or nose, for example
- objects driven into the skin by accident, such as fish hooks, splinters, or slivers of metal or glass
- objects which have entered the eye by accident, such as grit particles.

The history given by the patient or their carer is very important in indicating the type, size or quantity of foreign bodies which need to be removed. Assessment of each situation, including the patient, the history and the type and location of the object, will result in a different plan of care for each occasion. However, some general principles are:

- Foreign bodies in the eye can cause serious damage and should only be removed by a nurse with specialist training in opthalmic care, or by a GP.
- If a foreign body is not visible, e.g. is too far up the nose to be seen, then any attempt to grasp and remove it is likely to push it further in, and should not be made.
- Foreign bodies in the nose or throat are in danger of being inhaled if dislodged, and should be referred for the attention of the patient's GP, who may refer to an ear, nose and throat specialist.
- Foreign bodies in the ear can often be seen using an auriscope and removed with fine-toothed forceps or by syringing.
- Some useful instruments and methods for removing foreign bodies are shown in Table 20.2.

> ⚠️ **If there is any doubt that all foreign bodies have been removed, then the patient's GP may refer for X-ray or other diagnostic investigation.**

Table 20.2
Instruments and methods for removal of some foreign bodies (FBs)

Instrument/method of removal	Suitable for
Fine forceps	Visible small FBs in ears or nose (e.g. beads, plastic toys) Larger splinters of wood or glass in skin Fish hooks in skin
Sponge-holding forceps	Objects visible in the vagina, e.g. forgotten tampon
Electronic ear syringing machine	Small FBs or particles of grit in the ear, smooth, difficult to grasp objects, e.g. beads in the ear
Sterile needle	Small splinters in the skin, particles of dirt or grit in abrasions

When the foreign body has been removed, it may leave a wound which needs to be assessed and treated following the principles described under 'minor traumatic wounds', above. Following removal of some foreign bodies, and particularly if they have been in place for some time (e.g. a forgotten tampon), antibiotics may need to be prescribed to treat infection.

PRESSURE SORES

Pressure sores (decubitus ulcers) occur when body tissue is damaged by unrelieved pressure. The commonest sites for pressure sores are where skin is stretched tightly over bony prominences which are subject to pressure. Examples are:

- the sacrum
- the heels and ankle bones
- the elbows
- the sides of the knees.

Pressure sores may develop through four stages:

- redness of intact skin
- partial-thickness skin loss (shallow crater)

- full-thickness skin loss including loss of subcutaneous tissue (deep crater)
- full-thickness skin loss with damage to muscle and possibly involving bone.

In addition to unrelieved pressure, shearing injuries to the skin, caused by dragging over sheets for example, may precipitate the development of a sore.

> ⚠ **It is essential that everyone who cares for a dependent person, including family and informal carers, is aware of the possibility of damage to skin caused by inappropriate attempts to change position. Good moving and handling techniques, and equipment to assist in moving if necessary, will minimize risk.**

There are a number of different risk assessment scoring systems used to predict the likelihood of a pressure sore in a vulnerable individual, including the Norton Scale and the Waterlow Risk Assessment Scale (see Table 20.3). Such systems have been criticized for a lack of validity and specificity but they emphasize the importance of an overall assessment of the individual.

Table 20.3
Tools for assessing the risk of development of pressure sores

Tool	Includes assessment of
Norton Scale	Mental status, incontinence, mobility, activity, physical condition
Modified Norton	As above, plus nutritional status, skin appearance, tone and sensation, and minus physical condition
Waterlow Risk	Nutrition, pain, reduced cardiac output,
Assessment Scale	effects of anaesthesia, plus weighting for female sex
Braden Scale	Sensory perception, activity, mobility, moisture, nutritional status, friction and shear

Prevention of pressure sores depends on:

- encouraging early mobilization, or active and passive exercises
- frequent relief of pressure by change of position, or mechanical means such as pressure-relieving beds or cushions
- good hygiene and skin care
- protection of skin from wetness caused by incontinence or inadequate drying after washes
- regular inspection for early signs of risk or damage
- modification of other factors which may increase a person's vulnerability, e.g. inadequate nutrition.

> **!** Every district has an equipment loan store from which specialized equipment for nursing people in their own homes may be obtained. Loans are usually organized through the community trust.

WOUND HEALING

The process of the healing of a wound – whatever its type or cause – takes place in three stages:

- the inflammatory stage
- the proliferative stage
- the maturation stage.

In the *inflammatory stage*, clotting takes place to stop bleeding, then the blood supply to the area is increased to bring macrophages and other cells to the injured tissue. These cells digest bacteria and devitalized tissue. They also stimulate the activity of fibroblasts, which rebuild tissue.

In the *proliferative stage* the fibroblasts produce collagen, forming a matrix to support new capillaries: the combination of collagen and capillaries is 'granulation tissue'. When the granulation tissue has filled the wound, epithelial cells migrate across the new tissue from the edges of the wound to cover the granulation tissue. This is known as 'epithelialization'.

In the *maturation stage*, collagen reorganization continues to strengthen the new tissue.

Healing can also be said to take place by:

- primary intention, or
- secondary intention.

Surgical wounds heal by primary intention: there is little loss of tissue, and the edges of the wound are held together by sutures. Pressure sores, leg ulcers and some traumatic wounds, which involve the loss of a quantity of tissue, heal by secondary intention. These wounds spend much longer in the proliferative stage, as there is much tissue to replace before epithelialization can take place.

PROMOTING WOUND HEALING

There are many factors which affect the rate and success of healing of a wound, apart from the dressing used. These include:

- underlying conditions, such as diabetes or immunosuppression
- nutritional status of the individual: protein, zinc, vitamin C and adequate carbohydrate intake help to promote wound healing
- infection in the wound
- drugs taken by the individual, e.g. corticosteroids
- blood supply to the area.

Each of these factors needs to be assessed for the individual, and a plan of care agreed which will remedy any deficits. For example, walking or special leg exercises may be recommended for a person with a venous leg ulcer to ensure good blood circulation to and from the area. It is important however to avoid short-term solutions where possible, if a change in lifestyle would be more beneficial to the individual

> ⚠ It is better to help an individual attain and maintain a normal healthy diet than to encourage supplementation at the time of injury or wound healing.

SUMMARY

Nurses in primary care deal with a variety of surgical and non-surgical wounds. A knowledge of the stages of wound healing, and factors which may accelerate or delay wound healing, is essential to both the assessment and treatment of each individual. As methods and dressings to promote wound healing are developing rapidly, regular training and updating in areas relevant to the nurse's work are an essential part of professional development.

References

NHSCRD 1997 Effective Health Care Compression therapy for venous leg ulcers. NHS Centre for Reviews and Dissemination, University of York

Department of Health 1996 Immunisation against infectious disease. HMSO, London

Wound care
Summary

246

21

Ear care

Most nurses working in primary care will be involved in ear care at some stage. Minor problems such as ear infections and impaction of wax are relatively common, and practice nurses see many people seeking treatment for these conditions. Nurses working with older people have a role in detecting and assessing hearing loss, as well as helping their clients to manage and maintain their hearing aids. Health visitors carry out screening tests for hearing loss in young children.

In order to carry out ear care in any setting, it is essential to know how to examine the ear, and how to recognize the different conditions which may affect it, as well as how to treat them safely and effectively.

AURISCOPIC EXAMINATION

An auriscope is a hand-held instrument for examining the ear, which incorporates both magnification and illumination. It is powered by batteries contained in the handle, and these and the small bulb in the head of the instrument may need to be replaced from time to time to ensure continued use. Plastic nozzles of varying sizes are supplied with each auriscope, and these should be washed with hot water after use.

It is impossible to visualize the tympanic membrane (ear drum) without the use of an auriscope, and as such examination is necessary before any diagnosis is reached or treatment undertaken, all nurses dealing with ear care need to know how to use an auriscope.

The instrument is held in one hand, while the other hand is used to lift the external pinna of the ear upwards and backwards to straighten the ear canal. The nozzle of the auriscope is placed gently at the entrance to the ear canal so that both the canal and the ear drum can be viewed through the magnifier.

> ⚠ It is important not to push the nozzle into the ear canal, as this can cause pain and impaction of ear wax, as well as limiting the view obtained.

Auriscopic examination may show

- a normal ear drum, pale in colour
- a perforated ear drum, or a scar from a healed perforation
- an injected (red) ear drum, sometimes tense, if the ear is infected (otitis media)
- brown or black wax fully or partially obscuring the view of the ear drum
- redness and swelling of the ear canal (otitis externa).

> **!** If the ear drum is perforated or injected, the individual should be referred to her/his GP for further assessment and treatment.

EAR WAX

The commonest reason for people to request ear syringing is ear wax which is impairing their hearing. The individual may have identified the problem, or, especially in older people, relatives may complain that hearing is deteriorating and ask for ear syringing to be carried out. As the procedure is frequently carried out by a practice nurse, they may make an appointment directly with the nurse, rather than being referred by the GP.

> **!** It is essential that the ears should be examined with an auriscope before ear syringing is carried out. Hearing impairment may be the result of another cause, such as infection, perforation or neurosensory loss, which may be either unaffected or exacerbated by syringing.

Ear wax consists of cerumen, a natural waxy substance, combined with shed skin cells, dust and other debris. It is a natural occurrence, and is usually discharged from the ear in minute quantities as part of the normal process of skin shedding and regeneration. However, it can occasionally become impacted deep inside the ear canal, especially if cotton buds or similar hard instruments are pushed into the ears to clean them. It only needs to be removed by syringing if:

• the individual complains of impaired hearing
• a clear view of the ear drum is needed, and is obscured by wax.

> **!** If pain, or a history of perforation is reported, ear syringing should only be carried out on the instructions of the person's doctor.

The equipment needed to undertake ear syringing is listed in Box 21.1. The procedure consists of the following stages:

Box 21.1   Equipment needed for ear syringing

- auriscope with variety of nozzles
- ear syringe or electronic ear-syringing machine
- bowl or receiver (preferably kidney-shaped)
- plastic cape and/or towel to protect clothing
- hand-hot tap water in jug or machine reservoir
- paper tissues to dry the ear.

- Prepare the patient by seating him/her and placing a towel or waterproof cape round his/her shoulders.
- Ask the patient to hold the bowl or (preferably) kidney-shaped receiver close to the neck on the side to be syringed.
- Re-examine the ear with the auriscope to confirm the presence of wax.
- Prepare a jug of hand-hot tap water, or fill an electronic ear-syringing machine reservoir with the same (see Box 21.2).
- If using an electronic machine, demonstrate the noise it makes to the patient before using it on the ear.
- Use one hand to hold the pinna of the ear upwards and backwards to straighten out the ear canal.
- Using the ear syringe or nozzle of electronic machine, direct a gentle jet of water towards the top and back of the ear canal (not directly at the ear drum).
- Observe the water returned from the ear for signs of ear wax, and examine the ear at intervals during the procedure to avoid unnecessary syringing once the ear is clear.

Box 21.2   The electronic ear-syringing machine

- This is an electric pulsed water action syringe.
- It consists of a reservoir for water, and a small motor which pumps the water in controlled pulses through a lead to a long hollow nozzle.
- The nozzle is used to direct pulses of water into the ear canal, aiming upwards and backwards.
- A variety of different-sized nozzles are supplied, all plastic, which can be washed and, if necessary, disinfected after use.
- The force with which the water is pulsed can be controlled by a variety of settings.
- It can be used to flush out foreign bodies from the ear canal as well as to remove impacted ear wax.

⚠️ **Ear syringing may be slightly uncomfortable, but should not hurt. If the patient complains of pain, stop syringing.**

Some people make regular appointments for ear syringing. It is important to examine the ears every time to check whether the procedure is necessary.

EAR INFECTIONS

Otitis externa – infection of the auditory meatus or ear canal – can be extremely painful and cause the ear to discharge serous fluid. Treatment may involve gentle cleaning of the area and the use of local wicks as well as systemic antibiotics.

Otitis media – inflammation of the middle ear – is also very painful, and the effusion in the middle ear, which may be serous, mucoid or purulent, causes the ear drum to become swollen and red. Systemic antibiotics are given, and, as children are often the sufferers, parents may need advice on reducing a high temperature and suitable analgesics for children.

'Glue ear' is a common condition in which there is a non-purulent effusion in the middle ear cavity. It is the most common cause of hearing impairment in children, though there is reported to be insufficient evidence to link glue ear with significant disability (NHSCRD 1992). The condition is of short duration and usually resolves spontaneously. In recent years there have been large numbers of surgical interventions for glue ear, including insertion of grommets and adenoidectomy, myringotomy and tonsillectomy. Authoritative guidelines now recommend a period of 'watchful waiting' on the part of GPs, to allow the condition to resolve spontaneously, rather than seeking surgical treatment for every case.

HEARING TESTING

Diagnosing, or raising the suspicion of, impaired hearing is an important function. In children, it should lead to further assessment and if necessary the provision of specialist treatment, or educational provision, so that effect on speech and language development is minimized, and social and emotional needs can be addressed. In older people, it should lead to specialist assessment for the provision of hearing aids which will maintain communication and prevent isolation frustration and depression.

The Health Visitor Distraction Test (HVDT) is a hearing test which is currently undertaken by health visitors with babies at 8 months of age. It involves two testers as well as the baby's mother, who holds the child. One tester holds the baby's attention by sitting in front of the child. The other, situated behind and to one side of the child, then uses a device to produce a sound of a known level of decibels. If hearing is normal, the child should turn to look for the source of the sound.

The HVDT was criticized in a report published in 1997, which suggested that the test identified less than 30% of children with a significant hearing impairment. The report proposed hospital-based universal neonatal screening, using an electronic ear probe, as a more effective and cheaper alternative (Davies et al 1997). Neonatal screening would not, however, identify children with acquired deafness, and it is likely that more than one screening method for children will continue to be used.

Audiology testing for the detection of hearing loss in children and adults is usually carried out in a specialist audiology department, although some general practices have equipment and trained staff to carry it out on their premises.

> **It is essential to know what your practice or trust protocols are for screening for hearing loss; hearing loss should never be accepted as inevitable and untreatable, even in old age.**

DEALING WITH PEOPLE WITH A HEARING IMPAIRMENT

Hearing loss affects 17% of people in the UK, and all community nurses will have contact with some hearing-impaired people in the course of their work. The Royal National Institute for Deaf People gives some practical advice for organizations and professionals who meet hearing-impaired people:

• Make lipreading easier by facing the person you are speaking to, making sure the light is not behind you, speaking clearly and keeping hands away from the mouth.
• Never shout at a hearing-impaired person: it distorts the lips for lipreading, and can be painful if they have a hearing aid.
• Find a quiet area to talk to someone with a hearing aid, as the aid amplifies background noise as well as speech.
• Do not try to talk to a hearing-impaired person from behind a glass screen, as the light reflected from it makes lipreading more difficult, and the glass itself muffles speech.
• Ensure that written information is available, in addition to verbal communication, when conveying important information; if using videos for teaching purposes, try to obtain ones with subtitles.

- Consider instituting a visual as well as an audible system for calling people in from waiting rooms.
- Keep names and contact numbers of sign language interpreters available for staff to use.

SUMMARY

Most nurses in primary care will be involved in ear care at some time, either in treating people with ear infections or impacted ear wax, carrying out screening tests or arranging for hearing testing when a deficit is suspected. People with a hearing impairment can be assisted to use primary care services more easily if some simple guidelines are followed.

References

Davies A, Bamford J, Wilson IA 1997 Critical review of the role of neonatal screening in the detection of congenital hearing impairment. Health Technology Assessment, London

NHSCRD 1992 Effective health care: the treatment of persistent glue ear in children. NHS Centre for Reviews and Dissemination, University of York

22

Infestations

Nurses in primary care will inevitably meet patients or clients with infestations. Such problems are relatively common, and it is essential that nurses can recognize them, and offer accurate and appropriate advice. Reports about the safety of some chemical treatments, for head lice for example, has raised public concern, and people expect health professionals to be able to give advice about this, and about alternative methods of treatment.

> ⚠ Although head lice and similar conditions are 'infestations', they are commonly referred to as 'infections', which sounds less judgmental, when speaking to patients or clients.

HEAD LICE

Head lice are a common problem. Up to 10% of primary school children may be affected in any one year, and the infestation can be passed on to other members of the family.

> ⚠ Although it is an infestation, the less emotive term 'infection' is often used about head lice.

The key facts to remember are:

• Head lice are wingless insects, approximately 2–3 mm long, which live, breed and die on human scalps. They can be seen as black specks on the scalp which move around. They do not fly or jump, but use powerful claws to walk from head to head during close contact.
• Nits are the empty egg cases of head lice. They appear greyish-white, and are firmly attached to the hair shaft close to the scalp.

> ⚠ Nits can be differentiated from dandruff because dandruff is dull, flaky and easily removed, while nits are shiny and firmly attached to the hair.

• The main symptom of head lice is intense itching of the scalp, as an allergic reaction to the bite of the lice. By the time itching is felt, the lice may have been living on the scalp for several weeks. Scratches on the scalp can become secondarily infected.

• Head lice can be detected by examination of the scalp for moving lice, or by combing out very wet hair over a pale surface such as a sink or piece of paper.

> ⚠ As head lice are dependent on the scalp for warmth and food, they cannot survive on hats, pillows or chair backs, and cannot be caught from these places.

• There are two common methods of treating head lice: by the use of special lotions which kill the lice, or by the 'wet combing' method, which physically removes them.

HEAD LICE LOTIONS

Lotions designed to kill head lice should only be used if live head lice or eggs have been seen on the scalp. Using them as a preventive measure, or 'just in case' is ineffective and allows resistance to develop.

There are various head lice preparations available by prescription and over the counter (see Table 22.1). It is important that parents or users are reminded to dry hair naturally when inflammable, alcohol-based preparations are used. Treatment with lotions should be accompanied by fine tooth combing for at least 10 days, so that dead lice are removed.

Some districts have policies advising the use of one preparation only for the treatment of head lice, to prevent the proliferation of resistant lice. Other districts have discontinued this approach. Some now operate a policy of recommending lotions only when the alternative 'wet combing' method has been tried, and there is evidence that live lice remain.

Table 22.1 Head lice lotions	
Name of lotion	Contains
Derbac M	Malathion 0.5%w/w
Full Marks	Phenothrin 0.2%w/w
Lyclear creme rinse	Permethrin 1%w/w Isopropanol 20%w/w
Prioderm cream shampoo	Malathion 1%w/w
Prioderm lotion	Malathion 0.5%w/w

> ⚠ Information on local policies for the treatment of head lice will be available from the community trust, or the health authority public health department.

Concerns about head lice lotions

Concerns have been reported about two substances found in head lice lotions: carbaryl and malathion.

Carbaryl, an organophosphate used in pesticides, was found to cause cancer in laboratory rats and mice exposed to high doses throughout their lifetime. The Committee on the Safety of Medicines has made head lice preparations containing carbaryl prescription-only items.

Malathion has also come under scrutiny, with a pilot study by the Health and Safety Executive showing that the levels of malathion metabolite in urine samples from people who had used the treatment were 5–10 times higher than in people occupationally exposed to the substance. Although further research is underway, this has caused concern amongst some parents and professionals.

THE WET COMBING METHOD

This method of treating head lice is an alternative to chemical treatments, which can be offered to families who are concerned about the use of chemicals, or when it is district policy not to use such remedies. The method summarized in Box 22.1. It works by combing the lice out of the hair while it is slippery with water and conditioners, making it hard for the lice to cling to the hair. It usually clears head lice over a period of 2 weeks.

Box 22.1 The 'wet combing' method of eradicating head lice

1. Wash the hair in the usual way using an ordinary shampoo.
2. Use ordinary hair conditioner liberally.
3. While hair is still very wet and covered with conditioner, comb through from the roots using a fine tooth comb. Ensure that the teeth of the comb slot into the hair at the roots with every stroke.
4. Comb out over a pale surface, such as a piece of white paper or a white sink.
5. Clear lice from the teeth of the comb after each stroke.
6. Repeat every 3–4 days for 2 weeks, so that lice hatching during this period do not have an opportunity to spread.

OTHER ALTERNATIVE METHODS

Some research has suggested that certain essential oils may be effective against head lice (Veal 1996). These include aniseed, cinnamon leaf, red thyme, tea tree and a blend of peppermint and nutmeg. They were found to be effective in a laboratory setting when applied in an alcoholic solution and followed by a rinse the following morning with a mixture of essential oil, vinegar and water. However, it would be difficult to justify recommending such treatments until there is more-clearly defined evidence of effectiveness and safety. Parents may want to consult a homeopath or other complementary medicine practitioner if they are particularly anxious to avoid using chemicals, and find that wet combing is unsuccessful.

> ⚠ If parents ask advice about consulting a complementary medicine practitioner, suggest that they should find one who is a member of a recognized and accredited association.

Other research (Magee 1996) has shown that parents sometimes use a range of inadvisable and sometimes dangerous practices to try to rid their child's head of lice. These have included using kerosene, alcohol and insecticides on children's heads, as well as head shaving. It is vital that all community nurses take every opportunity to promote safer ways of dealing with the problem of headlice.

SCABIES

Scabies is a mite (*Sarcoptes scabiei*) which burrows into the skin and lays eggs there. It is passed on by close and prolonged physical contact with an infected person, and is not likely to be passed on to professional carers. It causes intense itching, and the burrows of the mite can be seen on inspection, often in the web of the fingers or on the skin of the wrist.

Treatment for scabies consists of the application of an emulsion containing benzyl benzoate. This is available to purchase over the counter at pharmacies. It is applied after a hot bath, and must cover the whole body but not the head or face. The application is repeated after 5 days.

> ⚠ The emulsion needs to be diluted for children: the manufacturer's instructions must be carefully followed.

WORMS

There are a number of worms which can live in the human body, but the most commonly encountered in community practice is the threadworm, usually affecting children.

The worm enters the body as eggs in contaminated food, or can be picked up on fingers and later ingested due to poor hygiene practices. The eggs hatch in the intestine and develop into adult worms in 15–28 days. The adult females leave the intestine through the anus to lay eggs around the anal margin, causing intense itching, particularly at night. The diagnosis is usually made by a combination of:

- the intense anal itching, worse at night
- the presence of worms seen as small, white threads around the anus on inspection at night
- the presence of worms in the stools.

Threadworms are highly infectious, and the whole family of an infected person should be treated.

Worm treatments consist of piperazine or mebendazole, in liquid, syrup, tablet or powder form (see Table 22.2). Some consist of a single treatment, others recommend a second treatment to eliminate re-infestation from hatching eggs. Treatments can be prescribed or purchased over the counter from pharmacies.

Table 22.2
Treatments for threadworm infection

Name	Preparation	Treatment regime
De Witt's worm syrup	Piperazine	Treat for 7 days
Ovex (tablet)	Mebendazole	Single dose
Pripsen (powder)	Piperazine + senna	Take in milk or water; follow up dose in 14 days
Pripsen (tablet)	Mebendazole	1 tablet, chewed or swallowed
Pripsen worm elixir	Piperazine	Daily for 7 day repeated if necessary

> ⚠ **Mebendazole should not be used in pregnancy, so families which include a pregnant woman should be warned to ask for a different treatment.**

Practical advice to families with a person with threadworms should include:

- stressing the need for good handwashing techniques, particularly after having bowels open
- suggesting that the child wears pyjamas or pants at night, so that if scratching occurs, the fingers do not make direct contact with the anus.

SUMMARY

Community nurses are often asked for advice about infestations such as head lice, scabies and worms. They are common and simply treated conditions, but can cause families considerable distress. Concerns about the safety of some chemical treatments for head lice can lead to parents using inappropriate home remedies instead, and nurses need to be able to advise about safe alternative treatments.

References

Magee J 1996 Unsafe practices in the treatment of *pediculosis capitis*. Journal of School Nursing 12(1): 17–29

Veal L 1996 The potential effectiveness of essential oils as a treatment for headlice, *Pediculus humanus capitis*. Complementary Therapies in Nursing and Midwifery 2(4): 97–101

23

Minor surgery

Some minor surgical procedures have been undertaken outside of hospital settings for many years. Since the GP Contract of 1990, however, there has been a more organized expansion of these services provided through general practices.

Practice nurses have probably the greatest involvement in minor surgery carried out in primary care. Their responsibilities include both the care of the individual patient, the preparation and sterilization of instruments used in surgery, and often the organization of the practice's minor surgery sessions. These aspects of the role are described in this chapter.

MINOR SURGERY IN THE GP CONTRACT

Since 1990, GPs have been able to claim a fee for performing minor surgery in their practice. To be eligible, the GP must provide the local health authority with evidence of sufficient training and experience in order to register for the provision of minor surgery.

The kinds of surgery performed in general practice are shown in Box 23.1. The advantages to the patient of having such procedures performed in the doctor's surgery are:

Box 23.1 Types of minor operation carried out in general practice

- removal of
  - cysts
  - papillomas
  - foreign bodies
  - verrucae/warts
  - cervical polyps
- incision of
  - abscesses
  - infected cysts
- wedge resection of toenail
- injection of joints
- aspiration of synovial fluid
- electrocautery of warts
- cryotherapy of warts
- insertion of sutures.

- It can cut down waiting time, especially for the removal of dermatological lesions.
- It is usually closer to the patient's home, so more convenient for travel.

- The date and time can be fixed at the patient's convenience.
- The patient knows the doctor who will perform the operation.
- Any concerns which arise after surgery, such as bleeding, or painful sutures, can be quickly raised with the doctor who performed the surgery.

There are some conditions or circumstances, however, which indicate that a procedure should not be undertaken in a general practice setting, but referred on to a hospital specialist. Examples are:

- lesions which are suspected to be malignant
- lesions in difficult sites
- recurrent lesions
- lesions in particularly delicate places such as on the face.

PRACTICALITIES

Minor operations in GP's surgeries are either undertaken in specially arranged 'sessions', or more flexibly by adding one or two minor surgery patients to the end of a morning surgery, or before an afternoon surgery starts.

> ⚠ It is important that the appointments given allow sufficient time for each procedure, so that people do not wait a long time for their turn, and do not feel rushed out of the surgery afterwards.

It is useful to have an area of the waiting room where people can take time to recover before leaving the surgery. For some operations, it is best to ask the person, when booking the appointment, to arrange for someone to accompany them to the surgery, or at least to collect them afterwards.

In order to undertake minor surgery, the practice must have available:

- a range of appropriate instruments and other resources (see Box 23.2)
- a means of sterilizing instruments, or a supplier of single-use sterile instruments
- a protocol for obtaining patient consent for surgery (see Box 23.3)
- laboratory specimen containers and transport to appropriate laboratories
- sufficient staff, time and room to provide a safe, unhurried, private environment for surgery.

Box 23.2 Examples of instruments and equipment required for minor surgery in general practice

Reusable instruments:
- toothed dissecting forceps
- dissecting forceps
- Spencer Wells forceps
- sponge holders
- blade handles
- needle holder
- scissors
- curettes
- vaginal speculae
- electric cautery
- silver nitrate pencil
- cryocautery

Single-use:
- dressing packs
- sterile gloves
- suture material
- prepacked needles
- prepacked sutures
- steristrips
- syringes and needles

Other:
- cleansing agent
- dressings
- local anaesthetics

Box 23.3 Example of protocol for obtaining patient consent for minor operation

Surgery protocol:
- full explanation to be given to patient by GP booking appointment
- explanation must include possibility of scarring when appropriate
- patient (or parent of patient under 16) to sign surgery consent form
- consent form must be present in patient's notes on day of operation.

THE ROLE OF THE NURSE IN MINOR SURGERY

The role of the nurse divides into three main areas:

- dealing with the environment for surgery
- dealing with the patient undergoing surgery
- assisting at the operation.

Environment
The environment includes the room and equipment to be used for the minor operation. Minor operations are frequently

undertaken in a designated treatment room, but can take place in a GP's consulting room. It is important that the room is private and the procedure will not be interrupted, both to protect the patient's privacy and dignity, and to minimize distractions for GP and nurse during the operation. The room must be clean, the examination couch preferably able to be approached from both sides, and there should be a good, adjustable light source. A trolley for equipment is very useful, but otherwise a clear counter top close to the couch can be used.

Sterile dressing packs are usually bought in from a pharmacy (or obtained by the patient on prescription), or from local trust sterile services department. Single-use instruments, such as stitch cutters, and sutures are also bought in, but reusable instruments are usually owned by the practice. It is usually the practice nurse's responsibility to ensure that instruments are sterilized between use (see below).

A number of different local anaesthetic agents are available for minor surgery, and these are usually bought in for use in the practice from a local pharmacy. Different agents are appropriate for use in different circumstances, and on different parts of the body (see Table 23.1).

Table 23.1
Anaesthetic agents used in minor surgery

Name	Suitable for
Lignocaine (0.5%, 1% or 2%) *Cautions: Not to be used IV; do not exceed maximum dose; use with caution in patients with cardiac and hepatic disease.*	Local infiltration of skin for anaesthesia; lasts 1.5 h
Bupivacaine (Marcain) (0.5%)	Longer procedures; lasts 4–6 h
Lignocaine with adrenaline *Cautions: not to be used when anatomical part is supplied by an end artery (e.g. fingers, toes, nose, penis, scrotum) because of risk of ischaemic tissue damage.*	Anaesthesia with reduced bleeding

> ⚠ It is essential that the nurse assisting at the operation identifies the name and strength of the local anaesthetic being offered to the doctor, as different agents may be needed for different patients in the course of a list.

Patient

Care of the patient includes ensuring that he knows what procedure is to be undertaken, and that he has had a full explanation from the GP before signing the practice's consent form. Since the patient will be going home, rather than remaining under close supervision as he would in hospital, it is also essential to ensure that he knows:

• how to look after the wound and dressing after the operation
• what to expect in terms of pain, swelling, discoloration of the wound or surrounding areas
• what painkillers or other means of relieving symptoms, such as rest or elevation of the part, he can use
• when he should return for a routine check or suture removal
• whom he can contact, in and out of surgery hours, if he has any concerns or problems.

> ⚠ It is better to discuss these points with the patient before the operation takes place, when he is feeling well, rather than afterwards when he may be distracted by discomfort or anxious to leave the surgery.

Before the operation begins, the patient must be made comfortable and safe on the couch. Only the part of the body to be operated on needs to be exposed, and if it is a limb or the head, it also needs to be supported in an appropriate position. A couch is usually safer than a chair, even if the operation site is easily accessible, such as a finger. If the patient should become light-headed or faint, she will be better supported on a couch.

During the procedure, it is important to continue to answer the patient's questions and check regularly how she is feeling. Some 'minor' operations are significantly stressful for the patient, and she may become nauseated, light-headed or even faint during the procedure. If this happens, the patient should be laid flat on the couch until she has recovered, and allowed to recover adequately before leaving the treatment room. She will need to be accompanied home by a friend or relative.

> **!** A patient should preferably not be left alone in a treatment room to recover after a minor operation. If the doctor or nurse is required elsewhere, the patient should be accompanied to the waiting room where other staff can observe her until she leaves the surgery.

Operation

During the operation the nurse will also be responsible for assisting the GP. This will include:

* preparing the operation site, by shaving the area for example
* opening sterile packets of dressings, gloves, instruments, sutures, etc.
* offering local anaesthetic agents, instruments and sutures at appropriate times
* assisting in the procedure by, for example, cutting sutures to a suitable length
* collecting specimens produced (e.g. biopsies, removed papillomae) in appropriate containers for laboratory analysis
* dressing the site at the end of the operation
* ensuring the recording and dispatch of, and later the return of results relating to, any specimens taken.

> **!** Some authorities on minor surgery recommend that all excised lesions should be sent for histological examination, in case of unsuspected malignancy.

STERILIZATION OF INSTRUMENTS

Multiple-use instruments which are owned by the practice for minor surgery must be sterilized between every use. This is most commonly undertaken on practice premises by autoclaving. The autoclave (properly known as a 'benchtop steam sterilizer') uses steam under pressure to raise the temperature of the instruments inside to a level, and for a period of time, sufficient to achieve sterilization. This is usually 134°C for 3 minutes.

> ⚠️ **If an autoclave is not available, ask a local infection control nurse (usually employed by the trust) about effective alternatives: some traditional methods of cleaning instruments do not achieve sterilization and should not be used for these instruments.**

In using an autoclave it is essential that:

- instruments are cleaned with hot soapy water to remove blood and other matter before sterilization
- instruments are put into the machine unwrapped
- instruments with lumens or cavities are not autoclaved (unless autoclave has a pre-sterilizing vacuum cycle to draw out air)
- porous materials such as swabs, gauze and towels are not autoclaved
- single-use devices are not autoclaved (MDA 1997).

The Medical Devices Agency guidelines for the use of benchtop steam sterilizers state that autoclaves should be tested daily to show that the operating cycle functions correctly, and these test should be recorded in a log book. In addition, weekly checks of the door seal, security devices and pressure-limiting devices should be recorded, and a schedule of quarterly visits for testing by an authorized test person should be kept in the practice.

> ⚠️ **Any nurse involved in minor operations has a professional responsibility to ensure that patient safety is not compromised by inadequate sterilization of the instruments used.**

Other instruments used in minor operations, such as cautery machines, have their own requirements for cleaning, maintenance and sterilization. The manufacturer's instructions must be followed, and each nurse who uses them is accountable for the safety of the patient in doing so.

MINOR OPERATIONS PERFORMED BY NURSES

Nurses do not only assist GPs in performing minor operations. Some practice nurses, with appropriate training, undertake cautery or cryotherapy of skin lesions such as warts, and suturing of lacerations. The UKCC's 'Scope of Professional Practice' document makes it clear that nurses can extend their practice into this area provided that the conditions set out in the document are met.

> **!** All health care workers who undertake 'exposure-prone procedures' should be vaccinated against hepatitis B.

SUMMARY

There has been an increase in the amount of minor operations carried out on GP practice premises in recent years. Nurses involved in this work have responsibilities to ensure that the environment of care is safe and appropriate, and that patients have given written, informed consent for the operation, as well as assisting in or carrying out the procedures.

Reference

MDA 1997 The purchase, operation and maintenance of benchtop sterilisers. The Medical Devices Agency, London

24

Infectious diseases

Although immunization has reduced the threat of many infectious diseases, there are not many diseases which have disappeared altogether. Smallpox is one such, and the World Health Organization predicts that poliomyelitis will become another.

However, for the nurse in primary care, it is the commoner infectious diseases which concern patients and clients, and it is on these that the nurse needs to be able to give accurate and appropriate advice. These diseases can be conveniently divided into the traditional 'childhood' diseases, and others which affect adults as well as children.

CHILDHOOD INFECTIOUS DISEASES

The commoner childhood diseases, their causes and presentation, are shown in Table 24.1. Some of these diseases are potentially preventable by immunization under the national childhood immunization programme. These are:

- tetanus
- diphtheria
- pertussis (whooping cough)
- poliomyelitis

Table 24.1
Infectious diseases in childhood – causes and presentation

Disease	Cause	Presentation
Measles	Virus	'Cold', cough, pyrexia, conjunctivitis, 'Koplik's spots' (white spots inside mouth), red, flat rash spreading over trunk, head and limbs
Chicken pox	Virus	Pyrexia, blister-like spots scattered over trunk and face, typically at different stages (spot, blister, crust, scab)
Rubella (German measles)	Virus	Rash, often intense on face, raised lymph glands (post-auricular and suboccipital)
Mumps	Virus	Parotid swelling on one or both sides of neck, general malaise and pyrexia

- *Haemophilus influenzae* type B infections
- measles
- mumps
- rubella
- tuberculosis.

The schedule for the childhood immunization programme is shown in Chapter 14.

There are a number of reasons why a child may develop one of these potentially preventable diseases. The principal causes are:

- The child was not vaccinated (many areas of the UK achieve 95% uptake rates of childhood vaccines, but there are some pockets where uptake is less than 70%, leaving more than 1 in 4 children unprotected).
- The child was vaccinated but the vaccine was defective (e.g. vaccines which have not been stored at the correct temperature can lose their potency).
- The child was vaccinated but did not acquire sufficient immunity to ensure resistance to the organism (see Table 24.2).

When any of the above apply to children, a pool of 'susceptible' children is created who can be infected by the organism. The number of susceptible people necessary to create an epidemic of a disease depends on the infectivity of the organism: fewer susceptibles are required for an epidemic of measles, which is highly contagious, than of some other diseases.

OTHER CONDITIONS

One of the commonest presentations to community nurses and GPs dealing with children is the child with a rash. The

Table 24.2
Effectiveness of vaccines

Vaccine	Effectiveness
Hib vaccine	95%
Hepatitis B	80–90%
Influenza	70–80%
Measles, mumps and rubella vaccine (MMR)	90% (measles and mumps), 95% (rubella)
Meningitis A+C vaccine	90%
BCG (against TB)	70–80% (in studies of British school children)

Source: Department of Health (1996a)

parent often wants to be told which disease the child has, and how long they are infectious. Even with experience, it is often difficult to diagnose a child's condition from a rash and other non-specific symptoms, and the presence or absence of conditions such as measles can only be definitively proved by a blood test.

> ⚠ **It is particularly important not to suggest that a child has rubella without conclusive evidence, as this may give false reassurance about immunity in girls and lead to problems if they are exposed to the rubella virus during pregnancy.**

It is important to remember that there are other causes of rashes or spots in children, in addition to the common infectious diseases. Some of these confounding conditions are:

- other viral infections
- reactions, e.g. to bubble bath or soap powder
- rashes occurring as a known side effect of a vaccine such as MMR
- nappy rash
- bites from animal fleas
- heat rashes.

Often it is as helpful initially to advise parents on treatment of a hot, uncomfortable child as to establish a causal link with one of these factors. Box 24.1 gives some guidelines on advising parents.

Box 24.1 Advice to parents on dealing with children's rashes

- Bath child or affected part in tepid water rather than hot water.
- Dry by patting gently rather than rubbing.
- Use cotton sheets on bed rather than nylon or flannelette.
- Do not cover the rash with woollen clothing.
- Use calamine lotion on the skin to reduce itching.
- Prevent scratching by distraction or use of cotton mittens in young children.
- Give plenty to drink if the child also has a temperature.
- Ask pharmacist about antihistamine preparations which will reduce itching.
- Use a children's paracetamol preparation to help reduce the child's temperature.

Four major infectious diseases which have particular implications for nurses in primary care are:

- tuberculosis
- meningitis
- influenza
- acquired immune deficiency syndrome (AIDS).

TUBERCULOSIS

Tuberculosis (TB) usually results from infection by *Mycobacterium tuberculosis*, a bacillus spread by droplet infection. Three quarters of new cases are of pulmonary TB, diagnosed by the presence of the bacillus in the sputum. Non-pulmonary TB can be found in any of the major organs, but is not usually regarded as infectious.

Symptoms Symptoms of the chest disease include:

- cough with sputum production
- haemoptysis and chest pain due to pleurisy
- malaise, weight loss, intermittent pyrexia and drenching sweats (in miliary (widespread) disease).

TB is commoner in immigrant groups in the UK than in the indigenous population, and there is a higher incidence after return visits to the country of origin (JTC of the BTS 1990). It is also seen in homeless people, as well as those with impaired immunity due to AIDS.

Vaccine A vaccine against TB, the BCG (Bacillus Calmette-Guerin) was introduced for general use in 1953, and studies in British school children suggest that it is 70–80% effective (DoH 1996a).

Treatment Treatment for TB involves multiple drug therapy which must be taken over a period of months, to ensure effectiveness and reduce the likelihood of resistance to one drug developing. Multi-drug-resistant TB (MDR-TB) already exists and is very difficult to manage. Careful monitoring of people taking drug treatment for TB is essential, to encourage continued compliance and to identify the potentially toxic side effects of treatment if they occur.

Roles of nurses The roles of primary care nurses in the prevention and treatment of TB are varied and significant:

- School nurses test children for their immune status with regard to TB and help to deliver the BCG vaccination programme.

• Health visitors identify newly immigrant families who may arrive in the UK without having been immunized against TB in the past, and arrange for them to be tested for immunity.

• Specialist TB health visitors are involved in contact tracing and arranging testing and treatment for the contacts of someone who has been found to have TB.

• In areas where universal neonatal BCG vaccination is carried out, it is sometimes performed by midwives before the child leaves hospital.

• Practice nurses carrying out 'new patient' health checks in GP surgeries may identify adults who have not been immunized, and refer them on to a local chest clinic for immunization.

• Nurses working in residential or nursing homes supervise the drug therapy of elderly people who have TB through never having been vaccinated, or as a reactivation of an old infection.

• Nurses working with homeless people can identify those who show symptoms of the disease, help them to access appropriate treatment services, and to maintain an effective treatment regime.

In each of these roles it is important that nurses know the symptoms, prevention and treatment of the disease so that they can give accurate and constructive advice.

INFLUENZA

Influenza is a highly infectious, acute viral infection of the respiratory tract. It is usually self-limiting, resolving in 2–7 days. It can have serious complications, however, the most important of which is pneumonia. This is particularly serious in people with chronic conditions such as respiratory or cardiac disease. In the epidemic year of 1989, 25,000 additional deaths were attributed to influenza: in non-epidemic years it causes 3000–4000 deaths.

Symptoms   Symptoms include malaise, fever, headache and myalgia.

Vaccine   A vaccine against influenza is available (see Chapter 14). It has to be given annually as the vaccine changes each year to reflect changes in the virus. It is recommended for groups at particular risk from the complications of influenza, but not universally for the well population.

Treatment   Treatment of influenza is confined to treating the symptoms of fever, headache and malaise with simple analgesics, rest and an adequate fluid intake.

Roles of nurses   The roles of nurses in primary care are important:

- Practice nurses usually carry out influenza vaccination programmes every autumn (see Box 24.2).
- Nurses in residential and nursing homes ensure that their vulnerable residents have the opportunity to be vaccinated annually, by liaising with the GP surgery responsible for their home and arranging vaccination sessions.
- District nurses and health visitors may immunize elderly or chronically ill people on their caseloads as part of the practice-based vaccination programme.
- Nurses working with people with severe learning disabilities in institutional settings need to consider vaccination for their residents to prevent rapid spread of the disease.

It is important that nurses in primary care make every effort to identify people who would benefit from vaccination against influenza, and to give them information about the vaccine, in order to prevent unnecessary illness and death.

Box 24.2 A typical practice influenza vaccination programme

1. Practice identifies all patients in high-risk groups, from asthma, diabetes and coronary heart disease registers, through district nurses' caseloads and previous years' immunization lists.
2. A practice protocol is drawn up, indicating who will vaccinate patients, under what circumstances and in which premises, and nurses undertake training or updating as necessary.
3. Special 'flu clinics' are advertised in advance by posters in the surgery so that people who need the vaccine can book appointments.
4. Visits are arranged to all nursing and other residential homes on the practice list to vaccinate elderly or vulnerable people who consent to receive the vaccine.
5. Vaccine supplies, ordered in spring or summer, usually arrive in October in time for pre-winter vaccination programme.
6. Practice nurses, GPs, district nurses and sometimes other members of the team vaccinate the target groups and other appropriate individuals, either in specially arranged clinics, opportunistically, or during visits to patient's homes. For each person vaccinated, either an individual prescription, or a written direction from the GP covering a group of patients, is obtained in advance.
7. All immunizations are recorded in the individual's notes, and notes and/or the computer records are tagged to indicate that the patient should be offered influenza vaccination again next year.
8. The practice audits the vaccination programme to find out what percentage of its vulnerable patients in target groups received the vaccine.

MENINGITIS

There are a number of different organisms which can cause meningitis, including *Haemophilus influenzae* type B, which is the subject of the 'Hib' vaccine in the childhood vaccination programme. Meningococcal meningitis is a systemic infection caused by *Neisseria meningitidis*. Group B meningococci strains cause about two thirds of meningitis cases, with Group C causing most of the rest. Group A strains are rare in the UK. Meningococci are spread by droplet infection or direct contact, with an incubation period of 2–3 days.

Infants and young children have the highest incidence of the disease, but there has been an increase in the incidence of the disease in young adults, mainly with Group C organisms.

Symptoms Symptoms of meningitis include malaise, pyrexia and vomiting in the early stages, and headache, photophobia, drowsiness and joint pains. The typical haemorrhagic rash may appear later (see Box 24.3).

Box 24.3 Features of the typical haemorrhagic rash of meningococcal meningitis

- It is petechial (small red spots under the skin) or purpuric (blotches under the skin).
- It does not blanche under pressure – this can be demonstrated by pressing gently on the skin with a glass, through which the rash can be seen to persist under pressure.

⚠ **The onset of the disease can be fulminant, causing serious illness very quickly. As early treatment and referral to hospital is recommended, the patient's GP should be contacted urgently if meningitis is suspected.**

Vaccine A vaccine is available against Groups A and C organisms, but not against Group B organisms. It is not used routinely, but is recommended for close contacts of cases of meningococcal meningitis, and during local outbreaks. It is also given to people travelling to parts of the world where the risk of acquiring the infection is much higher than in the UK.

⚠ **Vaccination against meningitis is required by the Saudi Arabian authorities for people travelling to the annual Haj pilgrimage.**

Treatment Treatment of meningococcal meningitis is started as early as possible, with a dose of benzylpenicillin given by the GP before the patient is transferred to hospital. Contacts of the patient are treated prophylactically with rifampicin, and, if the case is shown to be Group A or Group C meningitis, then vaccination may also be offered to close contacts.

Roles of nurses The roles of nurses in primary care with meningitis is twofold:

- being aware of the symptoms of meningitis, so that anyone suspected to be suffering from the disease can be quickly referred on to their GP
- to vaccinate people as appropriate during an outbreak, or after a case has been diagnosed, or if they are travelling to an endemic area.

> **!** **It is important to remember that there is no vaccine against meningitis caused by Group B organisms, so it will not always be appropriate to vaccinate people after a case of meningitis.**

HIV AND AIDS

Acquired immune deficiency syndrome (AIDS) is caused by the human immunodeficiency virus (HIV). It is usually transmitted in one of three ways:

- through sexual contact
- through contaminated blood products
- from mother to child at birth.

Symptoms At the time of infection with the virus, there may be non-specific symptoms such as sore throat, joint and muscle pains and swollen lymph glands. However, following infection, AIDS is often symptomless for a period of years. The virus affects the T helper cells of the immune system, binding to the CD4 surface protein. As the number of helper cells declines, the effectiveness of the immune system is compromised and opportunistic infections occur. The CD4 count is therefore sometimes used, in combination with measurements of the viral load, to track the progress of the disease.

The commonest infections and other conditions affecting people who are immunocompromised by AIDS include:

Pneumocystis carinii pneumonia (PCP)
Kaposi's sarcoma (KS) – a normally rare form of cancer
viruses such as cytomegalovirus
oral candidiasis (thrush).

In addition, the virus can affect the brain, causing encephalopathy, and leading to dementia.

There is currently no vaccine against the human immunodeficiency virus.

Treatment Treatment for opportunistic infections varies depending on the nature of the organism or condition. Before any opportunistic illness is apparent, prophylactic treatment can be given to prevent or inhibit the virus from damaging the immune system. 'Triple therapy' or 'combination therapy' refers to regimes involving a number of different drugs, usually taken regularly over a long period of time, which aim to slow the progression of the disease by interfering with the ability of the virus to replicate itself.

Roles of nurses The roles of nurses in primary care vary with the stage of a person's illness:

• Practice nurses and GPs are sometimes asked to carry out HIV testing at the surgery, and later to collaborate with the secondary care specialist in the monitoring and management of individuals with HIV disease.
• Community mental health nurses may be involved in helping patients, their partners, carers and families to deal with depression, fear, anxiety or grief following diagnosis and through developing illness.
• District nurses will be involved in nursing more-dependent patients at home in the later stages of the illness, during palliative and terminal care.
• Health visitors or community children's nurses will be involved in practical and emotional support to families when a child is suffering from HIV disease.

> **⚠ Pre- and post-test counselling for people having HIV tests is a specialist skill (see Box 24.4); testing should not be undertaken by nurses who do not have training in this area.**

Box 24.4 Summary of the Department of Health guidelines for pre-test discussion on HIV testing

• Named testing should be undertaken with informed consent.
• Individuals should receive information about how HIV is transmitted, and the significance of both positive and negative results.
• There should be a discussion of the particular needs and interests relevant to the individual.
• Specialist counsellors may be required if the circumstances of the individual are complex and time consuming, and further discussion is needed.

Source: Department of Health (1996b)

Most districts have specialist HIV/AIDS services, where nurses can obtain advice, guidance and further information if they need it. There are also many active support groups and voluntary agencies who can contribute in practical ways to the care or support of a person with HIV. Genito-urinary medicine (GUM) departments of acute hospitals also have much experience of counselling, testing and treating people with HIV disease, and they are useful resources to which community nurses can refer people.

MINOR INFECTIOUS DISEASES IN ADULTS

Nurses in primary care are often asked for advice on the more common minor infections, such as:

- herpes simplex ('cold sores')
- herpes zoster ('shingles')
- tinea pedis ('athletes foot')
- plantar warts ('verrucae').

Herpes simplex

Cold sores are caused by a virus, which, once acquired, can remain dormant in the cells (usually of the skin on the edge of the lips) until resistance is lowered by an infection. It then produces a blister which scabs, crusts and heals, usually within 7–10 days.

Sufferers can be advised that various preparations are available over the counter at pharmacies to treat the symptoms of cold sores. Dabbing with surgical spirit or aftershave helps to keep the sore dry and prevent secondary infection.

Herpes zoster

Herpes zoster is caused by a reactivation of the virus which causes chicken pox. The virus lies dormant in the dorsal ganglion of a nerve, and can reactivate many years later. Characteristic vesicles appear along the line of a nerve, often on the body. Because they follow the nerve, they will be unilateral and stop at the midline of the body. Pain along the nerve can be intense and may require strong analgesia. The rash usually dries and heals within 10 days, but the pain may persist as 'post-herpetic neuralgia', and may require longer treatment.

Oral antiviral drugs are recommended for some groups of patients with shingles (BSSI 1995):

- those over the age of 60 years presenting within 72 hours of the appearance of the rash
- those with involvement of the opthalmic nerve, presenting within 72 hours of onset

• those with active herpes zoster affecting the neck, limbs and perineum.

> ⚠ **Some people may be unaware that oral treatment is available for shingles: nurses meeting sufferers in the categories above should refer them to their GP to discuss treatment.**

People with shingles can infect susceptible contacts with chicken pox: the infectious period lasts until the lesions have dried up.

Tinea pedis

Athlete's foot is caused by a fungal infection. It frequently appears between the toes, and can cause desquamation as well as itching and scaling. Various over-the-counter preparations can be bought to treat it. They are usually powders or sprays and are recommended for use on the feet and inside socks and shoes to prevent recurrence of infection. In addition, people should be advised to keep the feet clean and dry, particularly between the toes.

> ⚠ **For someone who is living on the streets, obtaining dry socks and adequate shoes, and the opportunity to wash, may be as important as treatment with antifungals.**

Plantar warts

Verrucae are caused by a virus. They appear, usually on the soles of the feet, as hard flat lesions which are sometimes painful to walk on. Various topical creams and impregnated plasters are available over the counter to treat verrucae, which can be very resistant and prone to recur. Verrucae can also be removed surgically by curettage or cautery, although this can be unpleasant for children. Treatment with liquid nitrogen is sometimes undertaken by GPs or specially trained practice nurses as a minor operation in the surgery.

> ⚠ **Children need not be barred from swimming when they have a verruca, providing it is covered by a waterproof plaster.**

SUMMARY

In spite of advances in treatment and prevention, infectious diseases are still common, and many people with major infectious disease are diagnosed and treated in the community. Nurses in primary care need to be able to recognize, advise on and participate in the treatment of these diseases. Minor infectious diseases can cause considerable concern and inconvenience to sufferers, and nurses need to be able to recognize these conditions and assist people to treat themselves appropriately.

References

British Society for the Study of Infection 1995 Guidelines for the management of shingles–report of a working party of the British Society for the Study of Infection (BSSI). Journal of Infection 30: 193–200

Department of Health 1996a Immunisation against infectious disease. HMSO, London

Department of Health 1996b Guidelines for pre-test discussion on HIV testing. HMSO, London

Joint Tuberculosis Committee of the British Thoracic Society 1990 Chemotherapy and management of tuberculosis in the United Kingdom: recommendations of the JTC of the BTS. Thorax 45: 403–408

Further reading

Department of Health 1995 Health information for overseas travel. HMSO, London

Porter JDH, McAdam KPWJ 1994 Tuberculosis: back to the future. Wiley, Chichester

Infectious diseases
Summary

25

Palliative and terminal care

Palliative care is

> 'active total care offered to a patient with a progressive illness
> when it is recognised that the illness is no longer curable, in
> order to concentrate on the quality of life and the alleviation
> of distressing symptoms within the framework of a co-
> ordinated service' (SMAC/SNMAC 1992).

Palliative care can last for years, and can be applied to any
condition, though it is often associated with cancer. Other
groups of conditions in which palliative care should be
available in the final months or years include:

- respiratory conditions such as chronic bronchitis,
  chronic obstructive pulmonary disease (COPD),
  emphysema
- cardiac conditions such as congestive cardiac failure
- chronic degenerative diseases such as multiple sclerosis
  or motor neurone disease
- conditions affecting a range of body systems and
  functions such as AIDS.

Even people who are receiving institutional care (in a
hospital, hospice or other care setting) when they die will
often have spent the majority of the last year of their life at
home, receiving palliative care from the primary health care
team.

TEAMWORK IN PALLIATIVE CARE

Palliative care is a multidisciplinary activity, often involving a
wide range of members of the primary health care team as
well as informal carers, social services and others.
Professionals with particular expertise in palliative care are:

- Macmillan nurses – specialist nurses who offer emotional
  support and advice to patients and families requiring
  palliative care; they do not give hands-on care, but can
  help other members of the primary health care team to
  manage symptoms such as pain, constipation or insomnia
- Marie Curie nurses – specialist nurses who provide hands-
  on nursing care for patients at home, often during the
  evening and night to allow relatives and carers to rest
- consultants in palliative care – medical specialists in all
  aspects of palliative care; they are relatively few in
  number, and not every health district will have someone
  in this post
- clinical nurse specialists in palliative care – these posts do
  not exist in all areas, but where they do exist, the
  postholder usually has a remit to teach other staff, advise
  primary health care teams and facilitate communication

and shared protocols between primary care, secondary care and voluntary or non-statutory organizations dealing with people who have a short time to live.

District nurses are also frequently involved in the delivery of palliative care to people in their own homes. They will undertake assessment of the patient's and the family's needs (for care, and for equipment to deliver care), provision of care, and coordination of other services and professionals as needed.

Social workers may be involved to help patients and carers identify other needs, and to coordinate services such as housing and help in the home when necessary.

Welfare rights officers can help a family or individual to identify and claim financial benefits to which they are entitled, which may be essential to allow someone to stay in their own home.

Other clinical nurse specialists, such as breast care or stoma nurses, or continence advisors, for example, may be called in as required to assist the team in maintaining a patient in comfort and dignity throughout the period of palliative care.

Occupational therapists carry out individual assessments, both in hospitals and in the home, and can arrange for some items of special equipment, such as stair lifts, bath handles or raised toilet seats, to be provided to assist the patient and family to manage in the home.

Volunteer workers can play a significant role in helping a person through the palliative stage of their illness. Often their care enables an individual to remain in their own home rather than be admitted to a hospital or hospice. They may provide practical help, such as cleaning or washing linen, or provide emotional support and advocacy for the patient. The 'buddy' system, operated by the AIDS charity Body Positive is an example of volunteers who form supportive relationships with an individual and act as their advocate with other statutory and voluntary services.

These different members of the clinical and non-clinical team all have different parts to play in delivering palliative care.

The National Council for Hospice and Specialist Palliative Care Services (1995) suggests some definitions for the way these people contribute to care of the individual with a short time to live:

• *The palliative care approach* aims to promote both physical and psychosocial wellbeing. It is a vital and integral part of all clinical practice, whatever the illness or its stage, informed by a knowledge and practice of palliative care principles, and supported by specialist palliative care.
• *Palliative interventions* are non-curative treatments, given by specialists in disciplines other than specialist palliative care, aimed at controlling distressing symptoms and improving

patients' quality of life: for example, through their use of palliative radiotherapy, chemotherapy, surgical procedures and anaesthetic techniques for pain relief.

• *Specialist palliative care* is the active total care of patients with progressive, far advanced disease and limited prognosis, and their families, by a multiprofessional team who have undergone recognized specialist palliative care training. It provides physical, psychological, social and spiritual support and will involve practitioners with a broad mix of skills, including medical and nursing care, social work, pastoral/spiritual care, physiotherapy, occupational therapy, pharmacy and related specialities.

PRINCIPLES OF PALLIATIVE CARE

The National Council for Hospice and Specialist Palliative Care Services give the following guidelines about the key features of palliative care:

• patient and family participation
• collaborative multiprofessional approach by health care professionals
• use of appropriate medications, tailored to each patient individually, given regularly to relieve and prevent symptoms
• continued regular assessment and support, with emergency back-up available 24 hours per day
• access and early referral to specialist palliative care services for patient and family support if needed.

NURSES' ROLE IN PALLIATIVE CARE

In delivering care according to these principles, nurses working with people in palliative care must:

• respect the patient's choices about treatment and care
• promote active palliation of distressing symptoms
• acknowledge the patient as an individual
• provide care via an interdisciplinary team
• direct care towards common goals established and agreed with the patient
• remain non-judgmental
• act as an advocate for the patient
• ensure that care is delivered to the highest standards
• recognize the limitations of individual team members and consult and refer as appropriate
(Bullen 1995).

> ⚠️ 'Our aim is to free the patient from any distressing symptoms, physical, emotional, spiritual or social, and to maintain life at its full potential' (Hanratty & Higginson 1994).

DELIVERY OF PALLIATIVE CARE

Key factors in the delivery of palliative care are that it should be:

- unhurried
- observant
- compassionate
- competent.

When talking to patients who are terminally ill and receiving palliative care, Hanratty & Higginson (1994) suggest three rules:

- Always tell the truth.
- Consider that patients, if they ask, have an absolute right to be told whatever they wish to know about their diagnosis and prognosis.
- Regard it equally as a right for patients not to have information which they are not seeking thrust upon them.

The range and nature of symptoms for which relief may be needed is shown in Box 25.1.

Box 25.1 Some symptoms which may need relief in palliative care

Physical:
- pain
- nausea/vomiting
- diarrhoea/constipation
- intestinal obstruction
- anorexia
- sore mouth
- fungal infections
- dysphagia
- incontinence/retention
- pressure sores
- skin irritation
- oedema/ascites
- dyspnoea
- cough/hiccough.

Mental:
- fear
- anxiety
- depression
- confusion
- dementia
- grief.

Social:
- isolation
- withdrawal
- loneliness
- boredom
- frustration
- anger.

> ⚠ **The experience of each patient will differ, not only from those of other patients with the same condition, but from day to day.**

It is essential that the patient's condition is frequently assessed, and that the effect of treatments designed to alleviate symptoms is monitored. Nurses working with patients requiring palliative care should never hesitate to ask for advice and assistance from other, appropriately qualified or experienced, members of the team.

DEALING WITH GRIEF AND BEREAVEMENT

Palliative care of the patient may end with their death, but nurses in primary care often continue to be involved with the bereaved family. If the family is registered with the same GP as the patient, this involvement may continue indefinitely. The family's needs for care and support in dealing with their bereavement may be met by the primary health care team, or may require referral to other sources of support and counselling.

People who have experienced the grief associated with the death of someone close to them are often described as going through four stages:

1. shock and disbelief, during which they cope with initial practical matters
2. denial, usually short-lived, during which they may behave as if the person were still alive, or believe that they have seen or heard the dead person
3. growing awareness, which may involve anger, depression, guilt and anxiety
4. acceptance, which often does not occur until the second year of bereavement, and may be delayed longer (Thompson & Meggit 1997).

These stages, while common, are not experienced by all bereaved people in this order, or chronologically, and the timescales for feelings of bereavement vary widely.

> ⚠ **Each bereaved person is an individual with an individual experience of loss and grief.**

Nurses can help bereaved family members by:

- allowing them to talk about the person who has died
- allowing them to be upset or cry
- listening rather than talking
- acknowledging the bereavement in future conversations or consultations.

It is important *not* to:

- avoid mentioning the dead person
- change the subject when they are mentioned
- try to hurry the bereaved person through the stages of grieving
- try to undertake bereavement counselling if not specifically trained to do so.

> ⚠ **Remember there are specialist bereavement counsellors in most areas, who have the time, expertise and experience to help people professionally.**

Most people do not need routine bereavement counselling. Some people, however, are at greater risk of experiencing difficulty in coping with bereavement. These include:

- relatives of a young person who has died
- people with low levels of trust and self-esteem
- people with previous psychiatric illness
- people with little support from others
- people who have had a very dependent relationship with the deceased person

(Working Party on Clinical Guidelines in Palliative Care 1997).

These people might benefit from referral to a specialist bereavement service.

ANTICIPATORY GRIEF

When a death is anticipated, individuals and their relatives may experience 'anticipatory grief', including some or all of the stages of grieving. Relatives or friends of patients receiving palliative care may display anger, denial, anxiety or disbelief, and this can make assessment, care planning and delivery more complex for the nursing team. Caring for the whole family, not just the patient, is particularly important in these circumstances.

> ⚠ 'The most meaningful help we can give any relative – child or adult – is to share his feelings before the event of death and allow him to work through his feelings, whether they are rational or irrational' (Kubler-Ross 1985).

SUPPORTING THE TEAM

There are many factors which can make the palliative care or death of a patient particularly difficult for nurses and other professional carers. For example:

- if it is the first death with which an individual has been closely involved
- if it mimics a past or anticipated death in the individual's family
- if there are similarities (e.g. in age, family structure or medical condition) with the professional or his/her family
- if there have been difficulties or constraints in the provision of care.

In any of these circumstances occur, an individual may be particularly affected by the patient's death. It is essential that members of the primary health care team are aware of each other's feelings and reactions, so that support can be offered to colleagues, both routinely and when it is especially needed. This support can take the form of:

- regular multidisciplinary team meetings
- clinical supervision sessions
- significant event audits.

Team meetings These are essential to the planning and efficient delivery of care, as well as providing support to staff working in emotionally demanding circumstances. They provide an opportunity for individuals to express their feelings, receive advice, hear a different point of view and realize that they are not along in finding some aspects of their role difficult, frustrating or upsetting.

> ⚠ Remember that any member of the team, however experienced or senior, can experience stress at work.

In order to make such team meetings productive, they should consist of at least three elements:

- a review of the needs of the patient and the current care
- a chance for all team members to express their views and feelings about the delivery of care
- agreement on a plan of action to modify or proceed with the care package, and to address the expressed support needs of staff.

Clinical supervision This can have many aims, and is implemented differently in different settings and Trusts. Most forms of supervision, however, include an element of reflective practice, and an objective to provide staff with an opportunity to receive peer support. Meetings with a clinical supervisor, whether one-to-one or in a group, provide an opportunity to express concerns or difficulties arising from the provision of palliative care, and to reflect constructively on them. Equally, when the provision of care has been exemplary and the patient's experience has been positive, clinical supervision sessions may provide a forum to share this with others.

Significant event audits These usually take the form of a team meeting, led by an external facilitator. An event which has been 'critical' in some sense – usually because it has been particularly stressful, or because it has raised concerns about standards or processes of care – is discussed and analysed. The important characteristics of such an audit are:

- that all members of the team participate
- that blame is not apportioned
- that the intention is to learn from the incident
- that action is agreed to ensure that undesirable aspects of the incident are not repeated.

> **!** It is very difficult for a member of the team to both facilitate and participate. Trained and experienced facilitators can usually be found within a Trust, health authority or local audit group.

SUMMARY

The provision of palliative care is a multidisciplinary activity involving the primary health care team in its widest sense. Respect for patients and their families is the starting point for care, which may have to address a wide range of distressing and difficult symptoms. There are medical and nursing specialists in palliative care from whom other nurses can obtain advice, training and support. In addition, there are various mechanisms through which team members can give and receive peer support in this demanding work.

References

Bullen M 1995 Palliative care. In: Hinchcliff E (ed) The really useful handbook for community nurses. Publishing Initiative Books, Beckenham

Hanratty J F, Higginson I 1994 Palliative care in terminal illness, 2nd edn. Radcliffe Medical Press, Oxford

Kubler-Ross E 1985 On death and dying. Tavistock, London

NCHSPC 1995 Specialist palliative care, a statement of definitions. National Council for Hospices and Specialist Palliative Care, London.

Standing Medical Advisory Committee and Standing Nursing and Midwifery Advisory Committee 1992 The principles and provision of palliative care, HMSO, London

Thomson H, Meggit C 1997 Human growth and development for health and social care, Hodder and Stoughton, London

Working Party on Clinical guidelines in Palliative Care 1997 Changing gear–guidelines for managing the last days of life in adults. The National Council for Hospice and Specialist Palliative Care Services, London

26

Complementary therapies

Complementary therapies of all kinds have grown in popularity and acceptance in recent years. Some are now recommended, and even provided, by GPs as part of the treatment of certain conditions, and there are health centres and surgeries which have complementary therapy practitioners working from the premises.

Nurses in primary care may be consulted by clients about these therapies, both when clients are well and wanting to promote health and wellbeing, and when they are considering alternatives to traditional medicine when they are ill, or offered conventional preventive treatment. A common example is parents seeking a natural alternative to vaccines, usually through homeopathy.

> ⚠ **The Council of the Faculty of Homeopathy strongly supports the immunization programme, and has stated that immunization should be carried out in the normal way using the conventional tested and approved vaccines in the absence of medical contraindications (DoH 1996).**

Other situations in which community nurses may be asked about, or want to discuss with clients, the use of complementary therapies are:

- in pregnancy and labour, when women want safe and effective forms of stress and pain relief
- in palliative care, when conventional medicines and treatments may be insufficiently effective, or unacceptable because of their side effects
- in work with families from ethnic minority communities, who may want to use traditional forms of health promotion and treatment
- in work with individuals whose personal or religious beliefs preclude the use of some conventional therapies or treatments.

Complementary therapies are often used in conjunction with 'allopathy' (traditional Western medicine), and a client' interest in or use of such therapies would not be interpreted as criticism, or a rejection of all other types of treatment. Practitioners of complementary therapies may themselves be health professionals, or may have training only in their therapy. In either case, they should work in conjunction with other professionals involved in the client' care.

> ⚠ The British Complementary Medicine Association Code of Conduct states that 'practitioners must not countermand instructions or prescriptions given by a doctor'.

TYPES OF COMPLEMENTARY THERAPIES

It is important that the nurse understands the meanings of the terms used, and can advise clients on making safe and informed choices about therapies. Some of the more common complementary therapies are described below.

Acupuncture   This is a system of treatment which aims to rebalance energy by inserting needles in points on the body's meridians (energy channels). Its origins are in traditional Chinese medicine. Acupuncture can be used to treat sinusitis, headaches, low back pain, digestive disorders, chronic menstrual disorders and addictive habits such as smoking, and as an anaesthetic for surgery. It is usually performed with sterilized steel needles, although 'acupressure' involves using the fingers to apply pressure to the acupuncture sites.

Chiropractic   This is a technique involving manipulation of the joints and spine, developed by an American osteopath, DD Palmer, in the 1870s. It aims to treat mechanical disorders of the joints and spine, such as slipped discs, strains and generalized back pain. It is also used to treat other conditions such as arthritis and rheumatism, migraine, headaches and asthma.

Homeopathy   This is a comprehensive system of medicine developed in the late 18th century by Samuel Hahnemann, based on the belief that 'like cures like'. Remedies prescribed induce symptoms similar to those of the disease, and aim to stimulate the immune system into response. It also uses the 'infinitesimal dose' theory, which contends that dosages of remedies are most powerful when given in the lowest possible concentration.

Naturopathy   Naturopathy consists of a combination of therapies including dietary treatment and hydrotherapy. It aims to promote health by restoring balance in the body and its function, rather than by treating specific conditions in isolation.

Hypnotherapy   The use of trance-like states to influence the mind and body for therapeutic purposes was developed during the 1700s after being demonstrated by Franz Mesmer. It works by channelling the unconscious resources of the subject to effect change in the body. 'Classic hypnosis' relies on an authoritative practitioner and a passive and compliant subject. 'Ericksonian hypnosis' (developed by Dr Milton Erickson in the USA) uses less direct suggestion, and attempts to stimulate the subject's own unconscious problem-solving capability. Hypnotherapy is often used for conditions such as high blood pressure, migraine, ulcers or skin diseases in which elements of anxiety, depression or tension play a part. It can also be used specifically to treat phobias, depression and addictive behaviour.

Shiatsu This is a Japanese therapy, developed from acupuncture and massage, which uses pressure on acupuncture points along the body's meridians. The practitioner applies pressure using fingers, palms, thumbs and knuckles, and sometimes other parts of the body such as elbows or feet. The aim of shiatsu is usually preventive, intended to balance energy flows and strengthen the vital organs.

Aromatherapy This is a very ancient form of therapy which uses essential oils, extracted from flowers, leaves, bark, roots and other natural substances. They are massaged into the skin, inhaled, or used in a bath. They have been used to treat rheumatism, pre-menstrual tension, poor circulation, headaches, migraines, stress, insomnia and skin problems, among other conditions, as well as to promote wound healing.

Reflexology This is a technique of touch which treats the body by putting pressure on and manipulating reflexes, or responsive zones, in the feet and hands which correspond to different parts of the body. It was developed in the 1920s and 1930s by Dr William Fitzgerald and Eunice Ingham. The massage is carried out using the hands, and its principal immediate effect is relaxation and improvement of circulation. It has been used to treat back pain, migraines, sinusitis, and digestive disorders, as well as for the alleviation of pain.

Alexander technique This is regarded as a skill (body awareness and coordination) which is taught to students rather than a therapy which is administered. It was developed by Frederick Alexander, an Australian actor. The teacher uses his or her hands to identify hidden tensions in the muscles and teaches simple movements to 'inhibit' harmful tensions and 'direct' natural posture and movement. It is a preventive technique rather than a treatment for specific conditions.

Osteopathy This is a system of 'manual medicine' which deals with structural and mechanical problems in the joints, muscles, ligaments and soft tissues. It was developed by Dr Andre Still in the United States, and uses manual pressure and manipulation. Osteopathy has been used to treat joint pains, arthritis and sports injuries, but also functional conditions believed to arise from problems with structure: respiratory problems, irritable bowel syndrome, headaches, digestive disorders, dysmenorrhoea and circulatory problems.

Therapeutic touch   This technique was developed by Dr Dolores Drieger, Professor of Nursing at New York University, in the 1970s. It is based on the premise that the body has systems of energies, which cause illness when they are in deficit or imbalance. They are 'rebalanced' by the practitioner's hands, which do not touch the body but perform sweeping movements about 15 cm above it, to redirect energy flows and smooth out imbalances.

Common to all these therapies is the emphasis on the whole person, including mind as well as body.

> **!** **Most of these therapies and techniques require specific skills training for the practitioner; a nurse intending to offer complementary therapies to clients must have the appropriate training to do so.**

THE NURSE'S ROLE IN COMPLEMENTARY THERAPIES

The nurse's role may include:

- giving information to clients about the therapies available, their benefits and limitations
- discussing the principles of different therapies to help clients make a choice which fits their beliefs and preferences
- directing clients to the professional organizations which regulate complementary therapies to ensure that they find a safe and competent practitioner
- searching for the evidence of effectiveness of complementary therapies on behalf of the client
- discussing with the rest of the primary health care team the role of complementary therapies in their different caseloads
- incorporating one or more complementary therapies into their practice, if suitably trained.

> **!** **Practising complementary therapies in the course of employment as a nurse should be discussed in advance with your manager or employer, and undertaken in accordance with Trust or practice protocols**

Nurses in primary care are frequently involved to some degree with complementary therapies. If they are to undertake therapeutic interventions themselves, they should have appropriate training and the approval of their manager or employer. All nurses should be able to assist clients to make informed choices about different forms of therapy, and to find safe and effective practitioners.

References

British Complementary Medicine Association 1992 Code of conduct and guidance to practitioners. The British Complementary Medicine Association, London

Department of Health 1996 Immunisation against infectious disease. HMSO, London

Further reading

Stanway A (ed) 1995 The new natural family doctor. Gaia Books, London

Jarmey C 1996 Thorsons principles of shiatsu. Thorsons, London

Nightingale M 1987 Acupuncture: an introductory guide to the technique and its benefits. MacDonald Optima, London

Downey P 1997 Homeopathy for the primary health care team. Reed Educational and Professional Publishing, Oxford

Complementary therapies
Summary

27

Continence

Problems with urinary continence are very common, with up to three million people in the UK affected, and they can affect all ages from young children to older people. Community nurses in all settings will work with people who have problems with continence, or people at risk from continence problems:

• Midwives begin the process of teaching women to strengthen their pelvic floor muscles after childbirth to avoid future continence problems.
• District nurses work with people whose bladder function is affected by chronic degenerative diseases.
• Practice nurses undertake well-person health checks and over-75 health checks, at which continence problems may be discussed.
• Health visitors advise families with children suffering from enuresis (incontinence while asleep).
• Nurses working in nursing homes for the elderly, and in residential homes for physically or mentally disabled clients, often care for clients with continence problems.
• The continence advisor is a clinical nurse specialist working across a whole district, taking referrals directly from individuals, or from other health professionals, for assessment and treatment of continence problems.

It is important for nurses to be able to help sufferers to understand the causes of incontinence, and to offer them referral as appropriate to their GP or a specialist nurse for the necessary investigations and treatment.

> **! Incontinence should never be treated as inevitable; specialist assessment and advice should always be recommended to clients.**

CAUSES OF URINARY INCONTINENCE

These can be divided into three areas:

• problems with the bladder
• other physiological factors which affect the bladder
• external factors.

Problems with the bladder include:

• detrusor instability – in which there is failure to inhibit the reflex contraction of the detrusor (smooth muscle of the bladder wall)
• atonic bladder – in which the detrusor has lost its contractility, causing incomplete emptying of the bladder
• urinary tract infection.

Other physiological factors which affect bladder functioning include:

- outflow obstruction – e.g. caused by enlarged prostate gland, or impacted faeces in the rectum
- weakened pelvic floor muscles (e.g. following childbirth)
- some drugs (especially those which relax smooth muscle)
- some endocrine disorders (e.g. diabetes insipidus)
- immobility.

Environmental factors which affect continence include:

- emotional and psychological factors
- availability of toilet facilities
- availability of help when needed to use toilet facilities.

> ⚠ **An individual's living conditions may have as much influence on their ability to maintain continence as physical factors.**

Different causes of incontinence may present in different ways (see Table 27.1). Once presented, a complaint of incontinence should never be ignored. The assessment required to establish the cause of incontinence and

Table 27.1
Causes and symptoms of urinary incontinence

Cause	Common symptoms
Detrusor instability	Urgency – need to rush to pass urine Frequency – passing urine many times during the day
Weak pelvic floor	Stress incontinence – on laughing, running or coughing
Urinary tract infection	Urgency, frequency
Atonic bladder	Passive incontinence – incontinent at rest, frequency, poor stream, post-micturition dribble
Outflow obstruction	Hesitancy – difficulty having started to pass urine, straining, poor stream, post-micturition dribble

identify suitable interventions and treatment will probably include:

- a full history of the incontinence
- a full medical, surgical and obstetric history
- an assessment of social, emotional, psychological, environmental and sexual factors affecting the individual
- recording of current medication
- physical examination, including rectal, vaginal, neurological, and abdominal examinations
- urinanlysis
- urodynamic studies, investigating pressure flows in the urinary tract
- continence charting over a period of time.

> ⚠️ **The assessment and investigation of incontinence is a complex, specialist process, and should be referred to the individual's GP and the continence nurse specialist.**

Some of the interventions or treatments which may be considered are shown in Box 27.1. If, after a suitable period of treatment and intervention, urinary incontinence remains a problem to the client, then continence aids, such as disposable pads, penile sheaths or urinary catheters, may be supplied.

> ⚠️ **These methods of containing the problem should be a last, not a first, resort, and should be used following the advice of a continence nurse specialist.**

Box 27.1 Possible treatments and interventions in treating urinary incontinence

- bladder retraining
- habit training
- pelvic floor muscle exercises
- pelvic floor surgery
- alterations to fluid intake
- treatment of other conditions
- drug therapy/alterations to existing therapy
- changes to environmental factors
- use of aids
- catheterization.

CHILDHOOD ENURESIS

This is usually defined as 50% or more wet nights in a 2 week period for a child over 5 years of age. (Nocturnal Enuresis Working Party 1998). The assessment of children with this problem often involves a multidisciplinary team including a psychologist and paediatrician. Guidelines for management include urological assessment, and the use of an enuresis alarm in some cases only. Desmopressin, as a nasal spray or tablets, may also be recommended for a period of 3 months, with referral to a specialist enuresis clinic if treatment is unsuccessful. The use of 'star charts', recording and rewarding dry nights, is recommended mainly for encouraging compliance with other treatments, rather than in isolation (Nocturnal Enuresis Working Party 1998).

> **!** The treatment of enuresis in children combines the specialisms of continence promotion and paediatrics. Unless you have specific training in this area, it is best to refer on immediately to appropriate specialists.

THE NURSE'S ROLE IN PROMOTING CONTINENCE

While assessment of urinary continence and the instigation of treatment is best referred to a specialist, there are many actions which could be taken by a general nurse working in primary care to promote continence and to encourage people to seek help for incontinence.

To promote continence:

• Include emphasis on pelvic floor muscle care when talking about health to women, especially but not only in the antenatal and postnatal period.
• Encourage clients living with acute or degenerative illnesses in their own homes to review the toilet arrangements before they have any difficulties, and adapt their toileting habits to maintain continence.
• Review daily routines in nursing and residential homes to ensure that help is available when needed to assist clients to toilet facilities.
• Advise clients about treating chronic constipation, which may go on to cause urinary continence problems.
• Anticipate continence problems which may be caused by immobility, surgery or medication, and help clients to plan ahead to deal with them.

To encourage people to seek help:

• Include tactful questions on continence in all well-person health checks so that it becomes a routine enquiry and makes it easier for people to ask for help or information.
• Display posters and leaflets in clinic and surgery waiting rooms, highlighting the problem and giving contact details for the local continence service.
• Use National Continence Awareness Week (usually around March) to display extra information about continence, or to arrange for talks to be given to local groups.

SUMMARY

Continence is a common problem, caused by a range of different factors, and most community nurses will have clients with continence problems. Assessment and the selection of suitable treatments and interventions are best carried out by specialist continence advisors, and general nurses should refer clients to their GP or direct to the continence service. All nurses have a role in the promotion of continence, and in encouraging people with problems to seek help and advice.

Reference

Nocturnal Enuresis Working Party 1998 Nocturnal enuresis: a strategy for management. In: 'Guidelines', Volume 4, February

SECTION 5

Emergencies

28

Anaphylaxis

Anaphylaxis refers to an anaphylactic reaction occurring in many tissues throughout the body.

 An anaphylactic reaction is a hypersensitive reaction to a foreign protein.

It can occur following vaccination, or in response to penicillin, other medications, or foodstuffs such as peanuts, in some individuals.

Anaphylaxis following vaccination is very rare, but it is unpredictable, and all nurses involved in vaccination need to be aware of the signs of anaphylaxis, and the steps they should take to initiate treatment and obtain medical help.

In addition, nurses in primary care who are not carrying out immunizations may encounter cases of anaphylaxis in children or adults responding to food hypersensitivities, or insect stings. By the nature of their work, these nurses may not be in health centre premises, and may not have access to the equipment and drugs which would be on hand if a patient collapsed in a hospital setting. It is even more important that they are confident of recognizing anaphylaxis if it occurs, and are aware of, and able to implement, local policies regarding emergency procedures.

RECOGNIZING ANAPHYLAXIS

- Anaphylaxis often occurs very quickly, but can be delayed up to 72 hours.
- General signs are collapse with pallor, limpness and apnoea.
- These are accompanied by tachycardia, angioedema (swelling of lips, face and tongue), difficulty in breathing (stridor, wheezing) and in swallowing and speaking.
- Skin may become red, with itchy weals, red around the edges with pale centres.

It is important to be able to differentiate between anaphylaxis and fainting or panic attacks.

The following symptoms usually suggest fainting or panic, not anaphylaxis:

- sweating, nausea, dizziness, ringing in the ears, dimmed vision

- choking and hyperventilation
- bradycardia
- strong central pulse
- jerky movements and rolling of the eyes
- rapid recovery (1–2 minutes).

> ⚠ **Very young children rarely faint, and sudden loss of consciousness at this age should be presumed to be anaphylaxis in the absence of a strong central (carotid) pulse.**

Following a faint or panic attack, the individual should remain lying down for 10–15 minutes with feet raised.

TREATING ANAPHYLAXIS

Treatment of anaphylaxis is as follows (DoH 1996):

- Lie patient in left lateral position.
- Insert airway if unconscious.
- Send for assistance but do not leave the patient alone.
- In *mild anaphylaxis/allergic reaction (slowly progressing peripheral oedema, or urticaria alone), treatment is oral antihistamines or subcutaneous adrenaline*, with nebulized salbutamol, oral or parenteral steroids and parenteral antihistamines if necessary.
- In *severe anaphylaxis (with cardiovascular collapse) intramuscular adrenaline should be given immediately* (see Table 28.1 for dosages)
- If no improvement is seen, adrenaline dose can be repeated every 5–10 minutes up to 3 doses.

Table 28.1
Adrenaline dosages for use following anaphylaxis

Age	Dose of adrenaline 1/1000 (1 mg/ml) by SC or IM injection
< 1 year	0.05 ml
1 year	0.1 ml
2 years	0.2 ml
3–4 years	0.3 ml
5 years	0.4 ml
6–10 years	0.5 ml
Adult	0.5–1.0 ml (the lower dose for elderly or those of slight build)

• Piriton (chlorpheniramine maleate) and hydrocortisone may be given intravenously by suitably trained individuals.

> ⚠ **All patients with anaphylaxis will need to be referred to hospital for assessment, and further treatment if necessary.**

NURSES' RESPONSIBILITIES

The responsibilities of nurses in possible anaphylactic reactions fall into four areas:

• preparation
• recognition
• initiation of treatment
• summoning additional assistance.

Preparation

Preparation for anaphylaxis means being prepared to treat such a reaction, wherever it occurs. Nurses in primary care carry out immunizations in a variety of settings including people's homes, schools, nursing and residential homes, clinics and doctor's surgeries. It is essential that in each of these settings the nurse has access to the equipment necessary to treat anaphylaxis (see Box 28.1) and the means to summon help.

Box 28.1 Equipment to treat anaphylaxis

On emergency tray:
• adrenaline 1/1000 (1 mg/ml)
• 1 ml and 2 ml syringes
• 23G and 25G needles
• airways (range of sizes)
• chlorpheniramine maleate ⎫
• hydrocortisone   ⎬ These are not
• salbutamol   ⎪ found on all
• aminophylline   ⎭ emergency trays

Other if available:
• nebulizer
• face masks and tubing (variety of sizes)
• oxygen
• IV cannulae

Where nurses travel to patients to give immunizations, such as in patient's homes, they will need to carry an emergency pack with them containing the necessary equipment and drugs. If the home or premises does not have a telephone, the nurse will need to take a mobile telephone to the premises.

Working from health premises, such as a health centre or GP surgery, does not guarantee that the necessary equipment is available or easily accessible. It may be stored at some distance from the treatment or consulting room, and may even be in a locked cupboard.

Before undertaking any immunizations, the nurse needs to know the exact location of emergency equipment, what is contained in the emergency store, and who is responsible for ensuring that it is all present and in date. When undertaking immunizations, it is preferable for the emergency tray to be situated in the room where the immunizations are taking place.

Preparation for dealing with anaphylaxis also involves having the necessary training and updating to ensure that the nurse can respond appropriately to an emergency situation.

> ⚠️ It is a pre-condition of the delegation of responsibility for immunization from a doctor to a nurse that the nurse has adequate training in the recognition and treatment of anaphylaxis.

Recognition

Recognition of an anaphylactic reaction requires adequate training, as described above, and familiarity with the important differences in presentation between anaphylaxis and fainting or panic attacks.

> ⚠️ Department of Health guidance (1996) states: At any age, if in doubt, treat the patient for anaphylaxis.

Initiation of treatment

Initiation of treatment will usually consist of moving the patient into the left lateral position, inserting the airway and, if medical help is not at hand, giving subcutaneous or intramuscular adrenaline. If nurses are concerned about giving adrenaline in the absence of a medical colleague, they should ensure that the Department of Health guidelines on the treatment of anaphylaxis, listed above, are incorporated into a Trust or practice protocol covering their responsibilities in emergency situations.

> **⚠ Remember that the Code of Professional Conduct states that a nurse should 'act always in such a manner as to promote and safeguard the interests and well-being of patients and clients' and 'ensure that no action or omission on your part ... is detrimental to the interests, condition or safety of patients'.**

Following this initiation of treatment, if further medical, nursing or other skilled assistance has arrived, the nurse on the scene can prepare further injections (of chlorpheniramine or hydrocortisone), for administration by a suitably qualified person, and set up nebulizer equipment (if available) for the administration of salbutamol or other bronchodilating drugs.

Summoning additional assistance

Summoning additional assistance is an urgent early action, but must be undertaken without leaving the patient alone. In the case of a child, the parent or other carer accompanying the child could be sent to summon help, but might be too distressed to cooperate. In a nursing home or residential home, or at school, there will usually be other staff in the vicinity who can call for medical assistance. Some health centre or surgery premises will have a panic button, or agreed alert system which can be used to summon assistance: for example, repeated use of a buzzer.

It is essential that people responding to the initial call for assistance summon medical help to the scene. The intravenous drugs which may be necessary if there is no rapid response to adrenaline can only be administered by a doctor or trained paramedic, and as the patient's condition can deteriorate very quickly, they need to arrive at the scene as soon as possible after the collapse.

Other people who may respond, such as clerical or support staff, can help by clearing space around the collapsed patient, dealing with distressed relatives, directing doctors and other paramedical staff to the scene, and ensuring that all emergency equipment is in the room and ready for use.

After the emergency

After an episode of anaphylaxis, it is important to:

- replenish the emergency tray and replace emergency equipment

• review the episode to identify aspects of the response to the emergency which worked well and those which could be improved; a checklist of questions for the review is shown in Box 28.2.

Box 28.2 Questions to ask in reviewing the emergency

• How quickly was the reaction recognized?
• How easy was it to summon help?
• How easy was it to use the emergency equipment?
• Was everything necessary easily available?
• Could the emergency equipment be arranged more appropriately?
• Was enough assistance available?
• How well were the relatives and carers looked after?
• Did the protocol cover all aspects of the emergency?
• Are there any additional staff training or updating needs?
• Do any of the staff need additional support and debriefing?

SUMMARY

Anaphylaxis can occur, rarely, following immunization, or as a result of a hypersensitive reaction to a food or drug. It is essential that nurses are trained to distinguish anaphylaxis from fainting and panic attacks, and to respond appropriately in each case. Nurses in primary care have an additional responsibility to ensure that they have all the equipment needed to treat anaphylaxis in the various settings in which they undertake immunization, and that local Trust or practice protocols are in place to cover these situations.

Reference

Department of Health 1996 Immunisation against infectious disease. HMSO, London

29

Myocardial infarction

A myocardial infarction (MI) is the death of part of the heart muscle, the myocardium, from deprivation of blood. Community nurses may encounter an individual having an MI in any setting, including in the home, in a health centre, or on the street. As in anaphlyaxis, it is essential that they can

- recognize the condition
- initiate appropriate treatment
- summon assistance.

RECOGNIZING A MYOCARDIAL INFARCTION

A person having an MI usually experiences very severe central chest pain, sometimes but not always radiating into the jaw or arms. It is often accompanied by pallor, sweating, faintness, shortness of breath and nausea. There is tachycardia and hypotension.

> ⚠ **Some patients complain of less severe pain, or attribute it to other causes. A history of angina may raise suspicion that chest pain is cardiac in origin.**

It is often impossible to distinguish between an MI and severe angina without an electrocardiogram (ECG). However, if the patient has a history of angina, and has sublingual vasodilator tablets, they should be encouraged to take one immediately.

> ⚠ **As patient survival and subsequent health depends on early treatment, patients should be encouraged to seek assistance early rather than delay. Cardiac pain lasting longer than 30 minutes is more likely to be MI than angina.**

INITIATING TREATMENT

The treatment of severe chest pain which can be undertaken whilst awaiting medical assistance is limited:

• The patient should be made comfortable in a sitting or semi-recumbent position (not lying flat).
• A glyceryl trinitrate tablet should be given if the patient already uses them for angina.
• Pulse and blood pressure should be recorded if the equipment is available.

- The patient and any relatives or friends should be reassured that help has been summoned.

SUMMONING HELP

The patient's GP or an emergency ambulance can be contacted on behalf of the patient, and the decision as to which is most appropriate will depend on the individual circumstances. If the patient is on health service premises at the time of the attack, it may be quickest to summon a GP to the scene. However, if no doctor is on the premises, then an ambulance may be the quickest means of bringing skilled medical assistance to the patient.

> **!** **When starting work in a new area, always check the local Trust or practice protocol for such emergency situations; do not leave it until an emergency occurs to find out how and where to contact appropriate personnel.**

CARDIOPULMONARY RESUSCITATION

If a patient with a suspected MI becomes unconscious, check for evidence of cardiac arrest (i.e. no central pulse). If the patient does not respond to shaking or calling, remains unconscious with no central pulse, then cardiopulmonary resuscitation (CPR) must be started immediately:

- Transfer patient to a hard surface such as the floor if possible.
- Clear false teeth, food or other debris from the mouth.
- Begin cardiac massage and artificial respiration.
- If working alone, use massage and respiration in a ratio of 15:2. If working with another resuscitator, use 5 cardiac compressions to 1 breath.
- Mouth to mouth respiration can be carried out directly, but a Brook airway is often available at nursing homes, health centres or surgeries, and a face mask and Ambubag may be available at some centres.
- Check that a bystander or relative has summoned help, and, if available, send someone to direct the ambulance or doctor to the scene.

Dealing with a cardiac arrest in a public place or an informal setting such as the home is very different from dealing with it in hospital. There will be less specialized equipment available, none of the drugs, intravenous fluids or intubation options used in hospital, and fewer professionals to come to your assistance. However, there are sometimes trained first aiders, nurses or doctors amongst bystanders, particularly in big public events, and it is always worth appealing for such help as well as sending someone to telephone for an ambulance.

SUMMARY

An MI is a major cardiac event which can be difficult to distinguish from angina on clinical signs alone. Outcomes are improved by early treatment, so medical assessment and treatment should be sought as quickly as possible. The patient's history can be important in identifying whether they have vasodilator treatment to hand, and, if so, this can be used to try to relieve the pain. Other treatment is aimed at keeping the patient comfortable and under observation until emergency medical help arrives. If cardiac arrest occurs then cardiopulmonary resuscitation should be started immediately.

30

Acute asthmatic attacks

Asthma is a reversible airways obstruction which causes wheezing, cough, and difficulty in expiration due to muscular spasm in the bronchi.

It is a very common condition, thought to affect 10–15% of children and around 10% of adults. The disease ranges in the severity of its impact on individuals, with some patients only experiencing occasional wheezing, and others suffering severe attacks which can be fatal. There are currently around 1500 deaths a year from asthma. It is vital that nurses in primary care, who encounter people with asthma in a wide range of settings and age groups, can recognize the warning signs of an acute asthma attack, and take appropriate action.

RECOGNIZING AN ACUTE ASTHMA ATTACK

The British Guidelines on Asthma Management (1995) indicate some vital distinctions in the recognition of acute asthma attacks.

In adults the following factors suggest *acute severe asthma*:

- Patient can't complete a sentence because of breathlessness.
- The pulse is higher than 110 beats/min.
- Respiration rate is greater than 25 breaths/min.
- Peak expiratory flow rate is 50% or less of predicted or best reading (see Boxes 30.1 and 30.2).

In these circumstances the patient needs to be given oxygen 40–60% if available, nebulized salbutamol 5 mg or terbutaline 10 mg, and prednisolone or hydrocortisone by a doctor.

Box 30.1 Peak expiratory flow rate (PER)

- This is the maximum rate at which air can be expelled from the lungs.
- It is measured using a hand-held peak flow meter.
- An accurate reading depends on the patient's manual dexterity and coordination, and takes practice.
- Charts are available showing the 'predicted' peak flow rate for people of different ages in each sex.
- Comparison with predicted or best (i.e. best previous reading obtained by that patient, usually recorded in the individual's notes or their patient-held record card) is used to measure deterioration or improvement in condition.
- Patients in distress during an attack may be unwilling or unable to perform a peak flow measurement.

Box 30.2   Measuring the peak expiratory flow rate

In normal circumstances (i.e. not during an acute attack) the peak flow can be measured as follows:

- Stand up.
- Take a deep breath and release it.
- Take another deep breath and hold it.
- Holding the peak flow meter horizontally, seal the lips around the mouthpiece and blow out the inspired air as hard and fast as possible into the peak flow meter.
- Read the PER on the scale, then release the pointer so that it returns to zero.
- Repeat twice, and record the best of the three readings.

⚠ **If there is no response 15–30 minutes after nebulized salbutamol, the patient will need admission to hospital.**

Life-threatening asthma is present if the patient has:

- cyanosis
- a 'silent' chest (on auscultation)
- bradycardia or exhaustion
- a peak expiratory flow rate of less than 33% of predicted or best reading.

⚠ **A patient in this condition needs immediate admission to hospital by ambulance, with nebulized and intravenous drugs en route to hospital.**

The British Guidelines on Asthma Management also give indications on the recognition of acute severe and life-threatening asthma in children. In acute severe asthma, the child:

- is too breathless to talk/feed
- has a respiration rate of more than 50 breaths/min
- has a pulse rate of more than 140 beats/min
- uses the accessory muscles for breathing.

In life-threatening asthma, the child is:

- cyanosed with a silent chest and poor respiratory effort
- fatigued or exhausted
- agitated, or has a reduced level of consciousness.

> **!** The guidelines warn that children with severe asthma may not appear distressed, but the presence of any of these factors should alert to a possible diagnosis of acute severe asthma.

THE NURSE'S ROLE IN ACUTE ASTHMA

As an asthma attack can develop and a patient's condition deteriorate very quickly, it is essential that a medical opinion is sought as soon as possible. However, some practice nurses in particular often have specialist training in asthma management, and can play a part in starting treatment for an acute attack. Many GPs' surgeries are equipped with nebulizers, and keep bronchodilators as emergency stock drugs.

> **!** It is essential that an agreed surgery or Trust protocol exists if a nurse is to initiate treatment (e.g. nebulized bronchodilators) for patients suffering from acute asthma attacks.

Such protocols should set out:

- the clinical circumstances in which the nurse can give the named drug(s) to a patient
- the drug, dosage, frequency and route of administration (e.g. by nebulizer) of the drug(s)
- the training and updating necessary for the nurse to maintain appropriate knowledge about asthma
- the clinical or other conditions of the patient under which the nurse should refer the patient to the doctor or directly to hospital (e.g. all children, or patients with a designated peak flow level).

SUMMARY

An acute asthma attack can be fatal, and all nurses should be able to recognize such an attack. The usual course of action for the nurse is to obtain medical help for the patient as rapidly as possible, but some nurses, with special training and working under agreed protocols, may initiate treatment.

Reference

The British Guidelines on Asthma Management 1997 Review and position statement. Thorax 52(suppl 1): S1

Hypoglycaemia

Hypoglycaemia refers to decreased blood glucose levels: that is, below the normal level of 3.0–5.0 mmol/l. It is commonest in people with diabetes mellitus who have either too much (injected) insulin or too little carbohydrate to maintain normal blood glucose levels. It can occur in people with Type 1 (insulin dependent) or Type 2 (non-insulin dependent) diabetes.

Common precipitating factors for hypoglycaemia in diabetics are:

- a change in therapy
- a missed meal
- consumption of alcohol
- weight loss.

As with other emergency conditions, community nurses may encounter people with hypoglycaemia as part of their work, or coincidentally. Recognition and the initiation of treatment are the priorities.

RECOGNITION OF HYPOGLYCAEMIA

The first signs of hypoglycaemia are usually feelings of faintness and hunger, and tremor. These may be followed by slurred speech, confusion and aggressive behaviour. The patient is usually pale, sweating and restless. If untreated, hypoglycaemia may lead to coma.

> ⚠ **Some people with diabetes experience problems with a lack of warning symptoms of hypoglycaemia. A lapse into unconsciousness without the signs listed above does not mean that hypoglycaemia can be ruled out.**

If hypoglycaemia is suspected while the patient is still conscious, then asking about a history of diabetes will identify the probable cause for the symptoms. If semiconscious or unconscious, a relative or friend with the patient, or nursing staff in a care home, will be able to give a medical history.

Alternatively or in addition, measurement of blood sugar using a portable glucometer, available in most GP surgeries and health centres, and carried by some district nurses, will diagnose hypoglycaemia.

> ⚠ **An unaccompanied unconscious person may be carrying a card indicating that they are diabetic. A search of pockets, and the individual's wallet or handbag, might point to a probable diagnosis.**

TREATMENT OF HYPOGLYCAEMIA

If the individual is conscious, and able to cooperate, then he/she can be given a sweet drink such as juice or tea with sugar, to raise the blood sugar rapidly. Extra carbohydrate in the form of biscuits may then be offered in addition.

An unconscious person with hypoglycaemia cannot be given glucose orally. The usual methods of reversing a hypoglycaemic coma are:

- an injection of intravenous dextrose (given by a GP or after admission to hospital)
- intramuscular glucagon.

IM glucagon is usually available in GPs' surgeries, and diabetic patients may also keep some at home to be used by relatives in case of emergency. Glucagon can take up to 20 minutes to take effect, as it has to be absorbed from the muscle, and needs to be followed by some oral carbohydrate or sugars as its effect will wear off.

AFTER THE HYPOGLYCAEMIC ATTACK

Before leaving a patient, the nurse should ensure that the patient's blood sugar level is normal, and that they are aware of the need to continue monitoring their blood sugar reading, and to take adequate carbohydrate.

If IM glucagon has been administered, this should be recorded in the patient's record and reported to the patient's GP or other medical carer, so that a reassessment of their condition and treatment can be undertaken if necessary.

> ⚠ If the patient's own emergency supply of glucagon has been used, they will need a prescription to replace it as soon as possible.

SUMMARY

Hypoglycaemia is a relatively common and potentially dangerous complication of diabetes mellitus. Diagnosis is confirmed by measuring blood glucose levels. While the patient is conscious it can be reversed by giving sweet drinks followed by carbohydrate. If the patient is unconscious then IV dextrose solution, or IM glucagon will be necessary to restore blood sugar levels.

SECTION 6

Other activities

32

Patient/client advocacy

Advocacy is concerned with promoting and protecting the interests of patients or clients who are vulnerable and incapable of protecting their own interests.

As nurses working in primary care frequently have long-term relationships with their patients or clients, they are often asked or expected to act as advocates for them. Even in more transient relationships – such as between a nurse and a homeless person attending a drop-in clinic – there may be as great a need for advocacy as for physical or psychological care.

Some examples of nurses acting as advocates are:

- a nurse arranging with the breast-screening clinic for learning-disabled residents of a group home to receive invitations for screening
- a health visitor contacting a water company to avert disconnection of supply to a family with young children
- a practice nurse arranging for a GP to see a woman urgently for post-coital contraception
- a district nurse liaising between a housing officer and a homeless client.

> **⚠ While many community nurses work with a high degree of autonomy, those employed by a Trust should ensure that they consult their manager or team leader about the Trust's view of individual advocacy. Nurses working for GPs or private employers such as nursing homes may also need to seek guidance before spending time and resources on this work.**

WHEN PEOPLE MIGHT NEED ADVOCACY

Some groups of people with whom community nurses work and who might need advocacy are:

- people with learning disabilities
- people with severe or terminal illness
- people who cannot access services in the usual way (e.g. because they are not registered with a GP)
- people who have communication problems (e.g. illiteracy, poor English, sensory deficits such as deafness or blindness)
- people who are disadvantaged by poverty or discrimination.

Other individuals may need advocacy from a member of the primary health care team because their particular circumstances at a particular time make them vulnerable, or unable to act for themselves as they would at another time. Some examples are:

- women in labour
- people with an acute mental illness
- following bereavement
- during a family or personal crisis.

> ⚠ Advocacy is undertaken on request or when there is a clear need, in partnership with the client whenever possible, and always with the intention of passing responsibility, influence and control back to the client.

FINDING THE RIGHT HELP

The problems which such vulnerable groups might need help to address or resolve span a wide range from personal and social to financial or practical (see Table 32.1). Each case will be different, but a basic range of skills and resources is essential if a community nurse is to be able to act as an

**Table 32.1
Some issues on which advocacy might be needed**

Type of issue	Examples of problems
Housing	Unsuitable living conditions
	Homelessness
	Infestations
	Mortgage arrears
Access	Difficulty registering with a GP
	Lack of childcare for working parents
	Exclusion from screening programmes
Finance	Debt
	Unclaimed benefit
	Financial abuse of the elderly
Social	Domestic violence
	Isolation
	Discrimination
Occupational	Sexual harassment
	Industrial injuries/diseases
	Redundancy

advocate for patients or clients who need help. Some of the necessary skills are:

- the ability to discern the real problem, which may not be that presented by the patient or client
- the ability to empathize with the client, while remaining sufficiently detached to be objective
- communication and interpersonal skills to deal successfully with different agencies and individuals
- insight into personal limitations and motives
- ability to delegate, refer and work with others in the team, as few problems can be addressed by a single individual
- patience, tact and tenacity to pursue a long-term goal, as few problems can be solved quickly.

Resources which are necessary or desirable in this type of work include:

- use of a telephone and fax
- up-to-date directories of self-help agencies and support groups
- up-to-date local telephone directories
- key contact names and numbers for important local umbrella organizations (see Table 32.2)
- contact numbers for major national agencies (see Table 32.3)
- up-to-date leaflets issued by the Department of Social Security, the Department for Education and the Environment, the Post Office, and the major utilities such as gas, electricity and water companies.

> **⚠ Social security benefits change name, amount and eligibility criteria fairly frequently. It is better to refer people to their social security office or Citizen's Advice Bureau than to offer advice on entitlements yourself.**

SIMPLE STEPS IN ADVOCACY

In spite of the wide range of topics which may be the subject of advocacy work by community nurses, there are some logical steps which can be applied to most topics and give a framework for action. They are:

1. Take time to be clear about the issue, what it is, who is involved, what will be seen as 'progress' and what as 'success' by the client or client group, so that some goals can be set – otherwise a lot of time and energy can be spent on the wrong issue.

Table 32.2
Key local agencies

Type	Examples
Statutory	Local authority departments (e.g. housing, environmental health, education, social services) Benefits offices Health authority departments (e.g. Nursing Homes Inspectorate) Community Health Council Citizens' Advice Bureau Community Health Councils
Police	Community liaison officers Crime Prevention Officers Domestic violence unit/team
Employment	Jobcentres Disablement Resettlement Officers
Utilities	Local gas, electricity and water and sewerage companies
Other	Childminding coordinators Council for Voluntary Services Nursing and home care agencies Support groups / patients' groups Neighbourhood groups

2. Consult with colleagues and others, who may have dealt with something similar and may suggest either a solution or a short cut towards one – this avoids unnecessary duplication of effort.

> ⚠ Ask the advice of more experienced colleagues about topics or individuals which may give you particular difficulties.

3. Use local or national contacts to gain further information, identify options and test out responses.

> ⚠ Remember to be objective and tactful in your dealings with agencies and groups; it should be a collaborative attempt to address an issue rather than a battle.

Table 32.3
Examples of key national contacts

Type	Example
Statutory	Health Education Authority Department of Health Department for Education and Employment
Charities	The Stroke Association The Cancer Relief Macmillan Fund The Children's Society
Other	The National Council for One Parent Families The Patients' Association
Professional	The Community Practitioners' and Health Visitors' Association The Royal College of Nursing The Royal College of General Practitioners The Medical Defence Union

4. Keep in touch with the client, or group, passing on information and progress – the focus or importance of the issue may change and you may need to redirect your efforts.
5. When each of the goals set has been reached, or has proved to be unachievable, review with the client(s) and help them set new goals, if they wish, to which you and they can work.
6. If you have to pass over an issue to another professional, either because it is beyond your capability or because you are leaving that post, explain the situation to the client – don't leave it to another colleague to do so.

> ⚠ Advocacy depends on a relationship of trust, not only between the individuals but between the client and the whole service; if one professional damages that trust it can affect the client's subsequent relationship with others in the service.

WHAT TO AVOID IN ADVOCACY

There are a number of common traps for nurses engaging in advocacy for clients. While no-one can perform faultlessly at all times, it is worth trying to avoid the difficulties caused by:

- encouraging dependency, by taking on an individual's every problem
- overload, caused by taking on a whole range of different advocacy tasks at the same time
- distorted perception, by listening only to the client's view and not seeking the views of more experienced colleagues
- unrealistic expectations, from a client whom you have promised a solution
- burnout, from constantly battling with intransigent authorities, or bureaucratic agencies
- resentment, if clients do not appear sufficiently appreciative of effort made on their behalf, or fail to implement changes or solutions offered.

LOOKING AFTER THE ADVOCATE

Advocacy work can be very demanding and, even when some resolution or progress is attained, it is not always acknowledged. It is important that those undertaking this sort of work consider their own needs for advice and support. Some strategies which will help include:

- consulting colleagues, not only about the issues but about ways of dealing with them
- using clinical supervision sessions to reflect on and learn from the experience of advocacy
- sharing your experiences informally with colleagues
- acknowledging feelings of stress, frustration, resentment or anger when they occur.

SUMMARY

Many community nurses will have experience of acting as advocate for an individual or a group of clients, either regularly or occasionally. Being prepared with contacts, resources and a plan of simple steps can save time and effort. There are some essential skills which make advocacy most likely to be successful. The aim should be to create a three-way partnership between the client, the advocate and the organization or agency involved in the issue, rather than engage in constant battles. It is also important to find professional support for nurses undertaking advocacy.

33

Consulting the public

In recent years there has been much more emphasis on consulting users of the health service about health care. Often this has been confined to collecting complaints, or opinions about the way that health services are delivered, rather than inviting debate on key issues such as the allocation of scarce resources.

However, there have also been attempts to involve the consumers of health care more closely in the planning and development of services, principally through statutory bodies such as the Community Health Councils (see below).

Nurses in primary care are often involved in the initiatives to collect the views of users of the health services, because of their long-term relationship with and access to patients and clients.

METHODS OF CONSULTATION

Some of the common ways in which consumers are consulted about the health service are:

- through formal complaints procedures
- through informal comments/complaints forms
- through patients' panels, committees or participation groups
- through statutory bodies such as the Community Health Council
- through audits and research
- through national programmes such as 'Ask the patient'.

Formal complaints procedures

Formal complaints procedures underwent a major change in 1996, when a new three-stage procedure for all parts of the health service was introduced. This procedure is summarized in Table 33.1. A complaints system does obtain some useful views, although they are confined to a single incident. However, if lessons are learned from the complaint, and changes instituted to ensure that there are no future causes for complaint on the same issue, then complaints can be regarded as a limited form of public consultation.

Example: A formal complaint about a blood test result not passed on to the patient might instigate an investigation which shows that this was not an isolated incident in this surgery; an overhaul of the specimen-recording system and the protocol for giving results to patients might follow, and improve the service for all subsequent users.

Informal comments or complaints

Informal comments or complaints are often invited from the consumers of health care by notices and leaflets, or suggestion boxes, in waiting rooms and public areas of health centres and

Table 33.1
The NHS Complaints Procedure (from April 1996)

Stage	What happens
1. Local resolution	Complainant talks to someone close to cause of complaint (e.g. doctor or nurse, practice manager) or, if they prefer, to complaints manager of Trust or health authority Problem is sorted at this level if possible
2. Independent Review	If complainant is not satisfied, can ask Trust or HA to consider independent review. A 'convenor' will consider request, and if appropriate bring together a panel of three people – an independent lay chair person, the convener and one other – which will investigate and produce a report of its conclusions and recommendations. Report and letter from chief executive of Trust or HA re action to be taken as a result of recommendations are sent to the complainant
3. Ombudsman	If complainant is still dissatisfied, can ask Health Service Ombudsman to investigate

surgeries. The information gained from these exercises is often sketchy, but they can highlight areas of the service, premises or staff interactions, good or bad, about which comments recur.

Example: A number of comments praising the new system of calling people into the anticoagulation clinic by name rather than number might encourage other clinics in the same building to alter their systems in the same way.

Patients' panels, committees and participation groups

Patients' panels, committees and participation groups may exist in GPs' surgeries, community hospitals, group homes or other settings. They usually consist of volunteers, although the more organized may have some form of selection procedure. Their remit and purpose varies, with some seeing their role solely as fund raising and support, and others looking at some organizational issues such as appointment systems and visiting times. More vocal groups have sometimes been involved in lobbying on behalf of the practice or organization. Most groups do not consult their 'constituents' in any formal way, so their views may not be representative of the whole population of the practice, organization or area.

Example: A patient participation group at a GP surgery may lobby the health authority to try to prevent a new pharmacy opening in the area which would threaten the practice's in-house dispensing.

Community Health Councils

Community Health Councils exist in every health district. They were set up in 1974 to represent the interests and views of the consumer of health care, and to monitor health services. They hold public meetings, seek and pass on information to the public about local health services, and try to bring consumer influence to health authority decisions about service developments. The constituent members of CHCs are shown in Table 33.2. CHCs have the advantage of a statutory role in representing the consumer of health services, but they also have a large number of tasks to balance: monitoring quality in provider Trusts, monitoring planning and development in health authorities and consulting the wider public about current services and proposed changes.

Example: A CHC may hold a series of public meetings, attended by senior members of the health authority and local Trusts, as well as the public, to discuss alternatives for the provision of children's services in a district.

Audit and research

Audit and research can be used to try to obtain a representative sample of people's views about a particular aspect of health services. Audit usually compares performance against an agreed standard or set of standards: such as 'all clients should be able to register with a female GP if they choose' or 'eighty per cent of families should receive a visit from a health visitor within one week of requesting one'. Research usually aims to

Table 33.2 Membership of Community Health Councils	
Members	*Nominated by*
Chairperson	Appointed by Regional Office
18–24 other members	Half by local authority
	One third by voluntary organizations
	One sixth by Regional Office

find out something: such as the most useful services to offer homeless people from a mobile health centre, or the principal concerns of carers of patients with terminal illness.

Both audit and research usually involve efforts to find a representative sample of the population to be studied – by matching the study group with the general population for age, sex and ethnicity, for example. Alternatively, they may sample a whole population at a particular point in time (e.g. all patients being treated for leg ulcers during one designated month), or over the study period (e.g. the next 100 women attending the family planning clinic). These methods can often provide better representations of people's views than methods which rely on volunteer individuals, though they take longer to plan and to put into effect.

The method which can be used in audit and research studies to obtain the views of the selected sample are shown in Table 33.3.

Table 33.3
Examples of methods for audit and research

Method	Advantages	Disadvantages
Postal questionnaire	Can reach large numbers Relatively cheap Wide area sampled Quick to carry out	Generally poor return Poor response from non-English speaking/reading Excludes those with poor literacy Relies on lucid questions
Interviews	More information can be collected Questions can be explained More personal Includes people with poor literacy, or physical disability	Time consuming Requires special skills Interviewer can bias responses Can incur travel costs Excludes non-English speakers
Focus groups	Produce lots of info Generate discussion and exploration Take less time than individual interviews	Take time to arrange Require special skills Variety of data difficult to analyse and use

Example: A study of the views of 100 young people living on the streets might identify a list of major concerns with the health service which can be taken up with local GPs, community trust managers and social services to identify a common plan to bring the young people into mainstream services rather than providing a separate service.

'Ask the patient'

'Ask the patient' is an example of an organized approach to obtaining consumer views, which attempts to tackle the problems of populations with a high turnover and additional constraints such as limited language. The initiative was devised by the College of Health in 1992, initially to assess the quality of inner-city general practices, and combines several methods:

- a simple questionnaire
- observation by independent observers (such as CHC members)
- interviews with patients.

People were offered help to complete the questionnaires, and their answers were compared with the results of independent observation of the same aspects of service. This combination of methods may overcome some of the problems associated with the purely individual and anecdotal views obtained by some other methods.

The advantages and disadvantages of each of these methods of user consultation in the NHS are summarized in Table 33.4.

NURSES' ROLES IN USER PARTICIPATION

Nurses' roles may include:

- helping individuals to give their views (through advocacy, by giving information, or assisting in the completion of forms or surveys)
- planning initiatives to obtain people's views (designing audits or research, setting up user groups or panels)
- participating in eliciting and collecting views (by distributing questionnaires, identifying sample groups, running focus groups)
- introducing changes based on people's views (in their own work, or in the organization)
- reviewing the effectiveness of user consultation mechanisms in use in the area and recommending change when necessary.

Table 33.4
Advantages and disadvantages of different methods of hearing user views of the health service

Method	Advantages	Disadvantages
Complaints procedures	Thorough investigation produces useful information User has statutory rights	Focus on failure Reactive, not proactive
Informal comments	Reflect real issues for users Easy for consumers to use	Sketchy information Unrepresentative
User panels and groups	Informal and accessible Reflect real issues	Lack real power May not be representative
CHCs	Statutory support Part of structure of NHS	Large agenda May appear remote
Audit and research	More representative Can tackle more complex issues Makes recommendations or action plans	Takes longer to produce information May need skills training

> **!** Training on audit and research methods is often available free through the local health authority or regional office. They can also give contacts in local groups which aim to encourage and facilitate audit and research, and offer a wide range of help and resources.

THE FUTURE OF USER PARTICIPATION

The Government White Paper 'The New NHS – Modern, Dependable', published in 1997, introduced some major changes to the structure and functioning of primary care services and the health service as a whole. It also forecast greater user participation in planning and delivery of health services, nationally through an annual patient survey, and locally through the requirement for primary care groups to consult their local populations about services.

SUMMARY

There have been many different attempts to find out the views of the users of the health service, at levels from local GP practice to national surveys. Statutory bodies such as CHCs ensure that there is always a mechanism for representing the patient voice in the NHS. Enabling consumers of health services to genuinely participate in planning and decision making is more difficult than simply obtaining their views of existing or planned services. Nurses can be involved in helping people to give their views in a range of ways: from advocacy for an individual, to planning and executing major research projects.

Profiling and needs assessment

Profiling and needs assessment are sometimes used interchangeably to mean both producing a description of an area or caseload, and analysing that description to find out about the health needs of the population involved. It is useful to separate them, however, as each has a different aim and involves different skills and activities:

• The *profile* can be defined as a collection of data, both quantitative and qualitative, about an area, or a set of clients, and the services and facilities available to them. Its aim is descriptive, and it produces a tool which can be used as part of another piece of work, the health needs assessment.
• *Needs assessment* is the process of analysing that data, and other information, to define the factors which need to be addressed in order to improve health for that population. Its aim is to inform planning and service development, so that health improvements result from the changes implemented.

PRIMARY HEALTH CARE TEAM INVOLVEMENT

Community nurses such as health visitors, district nurses and school nurses have produced some form of profile, of their school or caseload, for many years. Practice nurses have in recent years begun to look at profiles of their practice in terms of the characteristics of its registered patients. The natural development from both these activities has been collaboration between all members of primary health care teams to produce profiles combining all the information held by each member of the team, and team efforts to analyse these profiles in order to plan ways to improve health.

PROFILES

The different kinds of profiles traditionally compiled by different community nurses are still undertaken, as they can inform planning for the individual's workload as well as forming the building blocks of a bigger profile (see Figure 34.1). These contributory profiles can be:

• caseload profiles
• practice profiles
• community profiles.

Caseload profile

A caseload profile is a profile of the individuals or families for whom a community nurse is responsible. A district nurse's

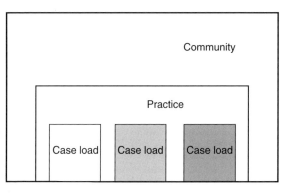

Fig 34.1 Profiles as building blocks.

caseload may change quite rapidly as people are discharged and new clients are referred. A health visitor's caseload is often more stable, although in areas where there is a lot of temporary accommodation, and families move on frequently, the turnover of the caseload will be much higher. Quite detailed information about caseloads can be assembled because of the manageable numbers of people involved, and the close contact between the client and the nurse. For example, district nurse caseload profiles can include information on client':

- age
- gender
- ethnicity
- housing
- financial difficulties
- dependency
- frequency of contact
- length of time on caseload.

A health visitor's caseload profile can include:

- size of households
- numbers of children per household
- single-parent families
- families with disabled persons
- families with children at risk.

To give a fuller picture of the context of care delivered to people on the caseload, this information is often combined with a description of the clinics and services available, the staff in the team and their qualifications and experience, and any constraints such as unfilled staff vacancies or increasing pressure on the service.

Practice profile

A practice profile is based on all patients registered with a particular general practice, so can include thousands of people. Information is usually less detailed about individuals, but can be aggregated to give useful information about groups. Information available from practice profiles can include:

- numbers of people in different ages groups
- numbers of people with different chronic conditions, e.g. diabetes, asthma or hypertension
- numbers of conceptions, births and terminations in the practice population
- child immunization rates
- uptake of breast and cervical screening rates.

This is combined with a description of the services and clinics available within the practice, the staff employed by and attached to the practice, with their qualifications and experience, and other factors affecting the practice. Commonly these include an assessment of the geographical and socio-economic characteristics of the practice area.

Community profile

A community profile includes these geographical and socio-economic factors for the whole area under consideration. It also describes employment, environment, services, demographics and other characteristics which affect the residents and their health. It generally deals with larger numbers than a practice profile, and draws on information collected on a large scale for other purposes, e.g. census data or the general household survey.

One of the difficulties in community profiling can be identifying the boundaries of the community, and finding data which matches the boundaries. Boundaries may be chosen by:

- electoral wards
- postcode areas
- social services areas
- localities defined by health authorities
- natural features such as rivers or greenbelt land
- artificial features such as motorways, major roads or industrial estates
- locally defined areas relevant to the local population.

Much of the publicly available information on an area relates to wards, census or health authority districts, and may need to be combined or interpreted to fit other areas.

WHY PROFILE?

A profile can be used for many purposes, and profiling can be undertaken for different reasons. Commonly it is undertaken to:

- form the basis of a needs assessment exercise
- identify priority areas for planning and development
- help managers to plan the deployment of staff and resources
- demonstrate the importance or effectiveness of a service
- help an individual practitioner plan her/his work
- substantiate a bid for more staff or resources
- foster good team relations between practice and attached staff
- form part of an academic assignment
- form the basis of a bid for project or development monies.

 It is important to be clear why profiling is being undertaken, as different purposes will require different information presented in different ways.

STARTING TO PROFILE

The steps to producing a profile can be summarized as:

- planning
- data collection
- data analysis.

 Health needs assessment using the profile will be a later step (see below).

Planning

Planning is essential before data collection starts, as it is frustrating and time-wasting to acquire data which cannot be used, or which has already been collected by someone else.

Plan:

- a systematic search for existing profiles (see Box 34.1)
- the boundaries of the profile – caseload, practice or a defined community
- which data to collect (see Box 34.2) – there are lots of tried and tested models which can be followed or adapted (see 'Further reading')
- who might be involved in data collection – other primary health care team members, health authority staff, practice or Trust information staff

Box 34.1 Where to find existing profiles

- practice library or manager's office
- community trust library
- community trust managers' offices
- University department of nursing library
- Health authority public health department
- Community practice teacher's records

Box 34.2 Sources of large-area information for profiling

- Public Health Common Data Set, produced by University of Surrey: comparative data by geographical area on demography, fertility, mortality and morbidity
- OPCS census data, summarized as Census Supplement to the Public Health Common Data Set: includes resident population estimates, numbers with limiting long-term illness, household overcrowding and amenities, elderly living alone, lone-parent families
- The Health Survey for England, commissioned by the Department of Health, first carried out in 1991: samples 17,000 people annually, from 1991–94 focused on cardiovascular disease
- morbidity statistics from general practice: report of practice activity from 60 representative practices, produced every census year: measures morbidity presenting to general practice.

- how the data will be analysed – by hand or on computer, by whom, and to what timescale?

Data collection

Data collection can easily become an end in itself. It is important to collect only what can be used, or additional information which contributes something extra to the profile. Qualitative data can be as useful as quantitative data.

> ⚠️ Remember to note sources of data so that they can be validated if questioned, and the same source can be used to compare differences in future profiles of the same area.

It is useful to judge the validity of the data as it is collected, by considering factors such as the date it was produced, and the source of the data. Census data, for example, may be highly reputable, but can be up to 12 years old by the time the next set of census data is available. Practice age – sex registers vary in their reliability depending on how frequently they are updated with new patients joining the list and others leaving.

Data analysis

Data analysis may require specialist help, particularly if it is to be undertaken using computer software. It is essential to have planned for such help before starting to collect the data. Simple statistical methods such as calculating percentages or averages, or presenting parts of the profile as pie charts or bar graphs, may well be sufficient for many purposes.

> **!** If numbers involved are small, or there is any question about the validity of the original data, it is not worth performing complex calculations.

HEALTH NEEDS ASSESSMENT

This is the step following the compilation of the profile, in which the information gathered is used to identify health needs in the population profiled. It includes an assessment of the factors discovered which may be adversely affecting health – such as poverty, lack of social support, existing chronic disease or low immunization rates. From these factors, and the characteristics of the population and their environment, some conclusions are drawn about the health needs of the profiled population.

Identifying health needs is a complex undertaking. 'Needs' can be defined in different ways: for example, as

normative needs – defined by professionals or experts
felt needs – defined by an individual or community
expressed needs – asked for by an individual or community
comparative needs – defined by comparison with another individual or community rather than existing in absolute terms.

Health needs assessment is therefore generally undertaken as a collaborative exercise combining different views and expertise.

> **!** The public health departments of health authorities have particular expertise in assessing health needs, and are easily accessible to primary health care teams for advice, support and information.

Most community nurses undertake some form of profiling, and are involved in the complex process of needs assessment. Profiling can be time-consuming and challenging, and is best undertaken as a team effort, following careful planning.

Further reading

Billings J 1996 Profiling for health: the process and practice. Health Visitors' Association, London

Appendices

PROFESSIONAL

UKCC publications:

- UKCC 1992 Code of professional conduct for nurses midwives and health visitors. UKCC, London
- UKCC 1992 The scope of professional practice. UKCC, London
- UKCC 1992 A guide for students of nursing and midwifery. UKCC, London
- UKCC 1993 Standards for records and record keeping. UKCC, London
- UKCC 1993 Complaints about professional conduct. UKCC, London
- UKCC 1996 Clinical supervision for nursing and health visiting, a position statement. UKCC, London
- UKCC 1996 Guidelines for professional practice. UKCC, London
- UKCC 1996 Reporting misconduct. UKCC, London
- UKCC 1997 PREP and you. UKCC, London

POLICY AND PRACTICE REPORTS AND GUIDELINES

- Department of Health 1997 The New NHS – Modern, Dependable. The Stationery Office, London
- Department of Health 1998 Our healthier nation: a contract for health. The Stationery Office, London
- Standing Nursing and Midwifery Advisory Committee 1995 Making it happen: the contribution of nursing, midwifery and health visiting to public health. Report of the Standing Nursing and Midwifery Advisory Committee. HMSO, London

PRIMARY CARE AND NURSING

- Health Education Authority 1997 Promoting health through primary care nursing. Health Education Authority, London
- James L, Sidell M (eds) 1997 The challenge of promoting health: exploration and action. Open University Press, Buckingham
- Leathard A 1990 Health care provision, past, present and future. Chapman and Hall, London
- Littlewood J 1995 Current issues in community nursing. Churchill Livingstone, Edinburgh

- Luker KA, Kenrick M(eds) 1995 Clinical nursing practice in the community. Blackwell Science, Oxford
- Newton P, Long S, Joesbury H, Mathews D, Usherwood T 1997 All together now: competencies in primary health care teams. A study by the Institute of General Practice and Primary Care, University of Sheffield, Sheffield
- Twinn S, Roberts B, Andrews S 1996 Community health care nursing. Butterworth-Heinemann, Oxford

APPENDIX 2: PRIMARY CARE PROFESSIONAL JOURNALS

Journals Include:

- Community Nurse (Macmillan magazines)
- Community Practitioner (Community Practitioners' and Health Visitors' Association)
- Complementary Therapies in Nursing and Midwifery (Churchill Livingstone)
- Handbook of Practice Nursing (Churchill Livingstone)
- Journal of Learning Disabilities (Churchill Livingstone)
- Midwifery (Churchill Livingstone)
- Practice Nurse (Reed Business Information)
- Practice Nursing (Mark Allen Publishing)
- Primary Care Management (Churchill Livingstone)
- Primary Health Care (RCN Publishing Company)

APPENDIX 3: USEFUL ADDRESSES

PROFESSIONAL

- UKCC
  23 Portland Place, London, WIN 3AF
- Royal College of Nursing (UK)
  20 Cavendish Square, London W1M 0AB
- Community Practitioners' and Health Visitors' Association
  50 Southwark Street, London, SE1 1UN
- Royal College of Nursing (Scottish Board)
  42 South Oswald Road, Edinburgh, EH9 2HH
- Royal College of Nursing (Northern Ireland)
  17 Windsor Avenue, Belfast, BT9 6EE
- Royal College of Nursing (Welsh Board)
  Ty Maeth, King George V Drive East, Cardiff, CF4 4XZ
- Royal College of Midwives
  15 Mansfield Street, London, W1M OBE

- The English National Board for Nursing, Midwifery and Health Visiting
  Victory House, 170 Tottenham Court Road, London, W1T 0HA
- The National Board for Nursing, Midwifery and Health Visiting for Northern Ireland
  RAC House, 79 Chichester Street, Belfast, BT1 4JE
- The National Board for Nursing, Midwifery and Health Visiting for Scotland
  22 Queen Street, Edinburgh, EH2 1JX
- Welsh National Board for Nursing, Midwifery and Health Visiting
  13th Floor, Pearl Assurance House, Greyfriars Road, Cardiff, CF1 3AG
- Health Education Authority
  Trevelyan House, 30 Great Peter Street, London, SW1P 2HW
- Health and Safety Executive
  Church House, Great Smith Street, London, SW1P 3BW
- Institute of Complementary Medicine
  PO Box 194, London, SE15 1QZ
- The King's Fund
  11–13 Cavendish Square, London, W1M OAN

ASSOCIATIONS

- Association of Carers
  20–25 Glasshouse Yard, London, EC1A 4JS
- British Diabetic Association
  10 Queen Anne Street, London, W1M OBD
- Macmillan Cancer Relief
  Anchor House, 15–19 Britten Street, London, SW3 3TZ
- MIND–National Association for Mental Health
  15–19 Broadway, London, E15 4BQ
- National Asthma Campaign
  Providence House, Providence Place, London, N1 ONT
- National Childbirth Trust
  Alexandra House, Oldham Terrace, London, W3 6NH
- Royal National Institute for the Deaf
  19–23 Featherstone Street, London, EC1Y 8SL
- Womens Nationwide Cancer Control Campaign (WNCCC)
  Suna House, 128–130 Curtain Road, London, EC2A 3AR

Index

Y